VEGAN AIR FRYER COOKBOOK

300 delightful vegan recipes to boost your health and lose weight. 21 days meal plan included.

Table of Contents

Introduction

The air fryer uses what is known as Rapid Air Technology. This technology allows it to cook food that would traditionally need to be cooked in deep fat. Unlike traditional deep frying methods, the food is not immersed in fat. Instead, it is cooked by circulating hot air. This air can circulate up to 200 degrees C. As you can imagine, such high degrees make it possible for the air fryer to cook foods such as pastries, chicken, fish and chips and so forth.

Just how awesome is that?

Think for a moment. It would take just one tablespoon of oil to cook some French Fries! Yes, the air fryer really is that awesome. But that's not the only thing that makes it awesome. The air fryer is also created to cook food faster, more efficiently and more appropriately. This is assured by its cooking chamber. The heating element is located closer to the food and this means the radiating heat is not wasted. The heat is allowed to do its work without deviations.

Additionally, the air fryer comes fully equipped with an exhaust fan. What does this do? As has already been stated, the air fryer cooks food via hot air. In order for this to work effectively, the air needs to circulate. This is where the exhaust fan comes in. It keeps the air moving such that the food is cooked evenly. The air is constantly circulating and passing through the food. Thus, everything in the air fryer is met with the same heating temperature. The simplicity of this undoubtedly makes the air fryer stand out.

But what about the high temperatures?

Yes, the air fryer uses superheated air to cook your food. This does not mean that you should be afraid of such high temperatures. The air Fryer's design makes it not only safe but also environmentally friendly. Each air fryer has its own coding system. This includes a fan that is carefully mounted onto a motor axis. This fan is the one that controls the air fryer's internal temperature. As a result, the internal environment is always clean and healthy.

All in all, the air fryer is not a complex appliance. All you need to know about it is that it has a grill and a fan. The grill provides the heat and the fan circulates the heated air. This results in foods that have a crispy outer layer but a soft inside. A dream come true.

Chapter 1 What is an Air Fryer?

An air fryer is basically a kitchen appliance that cooks food by circulating superheated air. This extraordinary appliance can roast, fry, grill and bake food with very little oil.

Benefits of An Air Fryer

There are loads of benefits when it comes to cooking with an air fryer. Here is a list of benefits that is sure to get you excited.

You can cook food really quickly in an air fryer.

It helps you cook exceptionally healthier fried foods as compared to the traditional frying methods.

Air fryers are very user friendly and easy to operate.

They are easy to clean and easy to maintain.

It uses much lesser amounts of oil while cooking without compromising on the taste of the food, thereby helping you to shed those extra calories without much effort and sacrifice.

Air fryers are much safer to use.

Brief History of The Air Fryer

Air fryers are relatively new to the market. They came into being only a couple of years ago in 2010, where they were first launched in Europe and Australia. They later made their way to the North American and Japanese markets.

Within a few years they have become an important part of the kitchen. In UK and Netherlands, this machine is mainly used to cook chips while in Japan it is mainly used to cook fried prawns. Americans began using it primarily to prepare chicken wings.

Chapter 2 Introduction to Vegan

What is Vegan?

Contrary to popular belief, vegan is not simply a type of diet.

It is actually a lifestyle that involves abstinence from the use of any animal products, not just food but any other product made from animal-derived materials (e.g. bags made from crocodile skin, jackets made of bear's fur and so on).

In this book, we will focus primarily on vegan diet, which is often confused with vegetarian diet.

In a vegetarian diet, the dieter consumes primarily fruits and vegetables and completely avoids meat, fish, seafood and poultry. However, the difference between vegans and vegetarians is that the latter still consumes animal derived products that are non-meat such as eggs, honey, milk and dairy. Vegans do not consume anything that is made of or by animals.

Why We Eat Vegan

Vegans have various reasons for adopting this type of diet.

Many do for health reasons.

In a report by the Academy of Nutrition and Diabetics, it has been shown that vegans are at less risk of many serious health conditions including cancer, heart disease, diabetes and high blood pressure, among others.

Research has also proven that vegans on average weigh 20 pounds lighter than people who consume meat. But unlike weight loss fad diets, this one produces long-term results and does not leave you feeling sluggish and weak.

Other vegans do this to save animals. Going vegan actually helps save up to 200 animals each year. This not only reduces the number of deaths but also prevents major sufferings in animal farms. Choosing plant-based food products is definitely the way to go for many animal lovers.

Guidelines and Rules for Eating Vegan

There are actually different types of vegan diets that you have to know about, and right away, you'll get the guidelines and rules for each one. They are quite simple and straightforward.

Whole food vegan diet

This vegan diet focuses on the consumption of whole plant foods including whole grains, legumes, nuts, seeds, fruits and vegetables.

Raw food vegan diet

This one involves eating fruits and vegetables and other plant foods that are raw and fresh, or are cooked at temperatures below 118 degrees F.

80/10/10 vegan diet

In this type of vegan diet, you will have to limit intake of plants that are rich in fat such as nuts, avocados, and so on. Instead, you will consume mainly fresh raw fruits and leafy greens.

Starch solution vegan diet

This refers to a low-fat, high-carb vegan diet that focuses on consumption of cooked starches such as rice, corn and potatoes.

Junk food vegan diet

In this type of diet, the person eats mock meats and mock cheeses, vegan desserts and other processed vegan foods.

It depends on you which one you should follow but basically, it would be a good idea to eat a balanced vegan diet. You can eat processed vegan foods occasionally but make sure that you also eat whole plant foods and fresh raw fruits.

What to Eat

Here's a list of the foods that you can eat:

Fruits and vegetables

Tofu, tempeh, seitan

Legumes (beans, lentils, peas)

Nuts and nut butters

Seeds (hemp, chia, flaxseeds, sunflower seeds)

Vegan milks and yogurts

Nutritional yeast

Whole grains, cereals

Plant foods (miso, kimchi, pickles, kombucha)

Mushrooms

Non-dairy milk (almond milk, soy milk, coconut milk)

Basically, anything derived from plants can be consumed in a vegan diet as long as edible and healthy. You can also eat food products designed for vegan diet (vegan butter, vegan cheese, and so on).

What Not to Eat

Here's a list of foods that you cannot eat:

Meat (beef, lamb, pork, organ meat, horse, veal)

Poultry (chicken, turkey, duck, quail, goose)

Fish and seafood

Dairy (milk, yogurt, cheese, butter, cream, ice cream)

Eggs

Any bee product

Any product with animal-based ingredients (egg whites, whey, lactose, casein, gelatin)

Remember, if the food product is from animal or created by animals, you cannot consume it if you're a vegan.

Tips for Success

Going vegan is not that easy. But here are tips on how you can achieve success with it:

Tip # 1 – Go slow

It may not be easy to suddenly shift to a meatless diet. Vegan is quite restrictive that you may find it difficult to adopt this diet at first. Don't worry. You can start gradually. You can start by first eliminating meat and meat products from your diet. Once you get used to it, then you can start avoiding other animal-derived products such as eggs, dairy and so on.

Tip # 2 – Don't succumb to pressures from people around you

People around you may not understand your decision to go vegan.

But you don't have to worry about what they think or what they say because this is your body, so it's ultimately your decision.

Also, you have to keep in mind that you're not doing anything bad, and that vegan diet is actually beneficial for your health.

Tip # 3 – Plan your meals

It helps to plan your meals by creating a weekly menu and listing down all the ingredients that you'll need to prepare these dishes.

Choose those that are easy and quick to prepare especially during times when you're busy so that you won't get tempted to go back to your old meat-eating ways.

Tip # 4 – Plan dining out

Eating at restaurants and at parties can be a challenge for any vegan.

Before going to a specific restaurant, check out if the menu has options for vegans. Go to restaurants that do have vegan menu selections.

If you are invited to a party, let your friend know that you have adopted a vegan lifestyle and that you will appreciate it if there are vegan foods that can be served for you.

Tip # 5 – Consider taking supplements

Going on a vegan diet may mean missing out on certain key nutrients that the body needs to thrive and be healthy. One example is vitamin B12.

Consider taking a supplement for this vitamin so that you do not end up becoming vitamin B12 deficient.

Be sure to consult your doctor first before taking any supplement.

Chapter 3 Snacks

1. Banana Chips

Preparation Time: 10 minutes

Cooking time: 10 minutes

Servings: 4

Ingredients:

4 bananas, peeled and sliced in thin pieces

A drizzle of olive oil

A pinch of black pepper

Directions:

Put banana slices in your air fryer, drizzle the oil, season with pepper, toss to coat gently and cook at 360 degrees for 10 minutes.

Serve as a snack.

Enjoy!

Nutrition: calories 100, fat 7, fiber 1, carbs 20, protein 1

2. Cabbage Rolls

Preparation Time: 10 minutes

Cooking time: 25 minutes

Servings: 8

Ingredients:

2 cups cabbage, chopped

2 yellow onions, chopped

1 carrot, chopped

½ red bell pepper, chopped

1-inch piece ginger, grated

8 garlic cloves, minced

Salt and black pepper to the taste

1 teaspoon coconut aminos

2 tablespoons olive oil

10 vegan spring roll sheets

Cooking spray

2 tablespoons corn flour mixed with 1 tablespoon water

Directions:

Heat up a pan with the oil over medium-high heat, add cabbage, onions, carrots, bell pepper, ginger, garlic, salt, pepper and aminos, stir, cook for 4 minutes and take off heat.

Cut each spring roll sheet and cut into 4 pieces.

Place 1 tablespoons veggie mix in one corner, roll and fold edges.

Repeat this with the rest of the rolls, place them in your air fryer's basket, grease them with cooking oil and cook at 360 degrees F for 10 minutes on each side.

Arrange on a platter and serve as an appetizer.

Enjoy!

Nutrition: calories 150, fat 3, fiber 4, carbs 7, protein 2

3. Tortilla Chips

Preparation Time: 10 minutes

Cooking time: 4 minutes

Servings: 4

Ingredients:

8 corn tortillas, each cut into triangles

Salt and black pepper to the taste

1 tablespoon olive oil

Directions:

Brush tortilla chips with the oil, place them in your air fryer's basket and cook for 4 minutes at 400 degrees F

Serve them with salt and pepper sprinkled all over.

Enjoy!

Nutrition: calories 53, fat 1, fiber 1.5, carbs 10, protein 2

4. Chickpeas Snack

Preparation Time: 10 minutes

Cooking time: 20 minutes

Servings: 4

Ingredients:

15 ounces canned chickpeas, drained

½ teaspoon cumin, ground

1 tablespoon olive oil

1 teaspoon smoked paprika

Salt and black pepper to the taste

Directions:

In a bowl, mix chickpeas with oil, cumin, paprika, salt and pepper, toss to coat, place them in the fryer's basket, cook at 390 degrees F for 10 minutes and transfer to a bowl.

Serve as a snack

Enjoy!

Nutrition: calories 140, fat 1, fiber 6, carbs 20, protein 6

5. Rice Balls

Preparation Time: 10 minutes

Cooking time: 35 minutes

Servings: 6

Ingredients:

1 small yellow onion, chopped

1 cup Arborio rice

1 tablespoon olive oil

1 cup veggie stock

Salt and black pepper to the taste

2 ounces tofu, cubed

¼ cup sun-dried tomatoes, chopped

1 and ½ cups vegan breadcrumbs

A drizzle of olive oil

Marinara sauce for serving

Directions:

Heat up a pan with 1 tablespoon oil over medium heat, add onion, stir and cook for 5 minutes.

Add rice, stock, salt and pepper, stir, cook on a low heat for 20 minutes, spread on a baking sheet and leave aside to cool down.

Transfer rice to a bowl, add tomatoes and half of the breadcrumbs and stir well.

Shape 12 balls, press a hole in each ball, stuff with tofu cubes and mold balls again.

Dredge them in the rest of the breadcrumbs, arrange all balls in your air fryer, drizzle the oil over them and cook at 380 degrees F for 10 minutes.

Flip them and cook for 5 minutes more.

Arrange them on a platter and serve them as a snack.

Enjoy!

Nutrition: calories 137, fat 12, fiber 1, carbs 7, protein 5

6. Tofu Snack

Preparation Time: 30 minutes

Cooking time: 20 minutes

Servings: 4

Ingredients:

12 ounces firm tofu, cubed

1 teaspoon sweet paprika

1 teaspoon sesame oil

1 tablespoon coriander, chopped

2 tablespoons coconut aminos

Directions:

In a bowl, mix paprika with the oil, coriander and aminos, whisk well, add tofu pieces, toss to coat and leave aside for 30 minutes.

Transfer tofu cubes to your air fryer's basket and cook at 350 degrees F for 20 minutes shaking halfway.

Transfer them to a bowl and serve as a snack.

Enjoy!

Nutrition: calories 90, fat 2, fiber 1, carbs 6, protein 1

7. Apple Chips

Preparation Time: 10 minutes

Cooking time: 15 minutes

Servings: 2

Ingredients:

1 apple, cored and thinly sliced

½ teaspoon cinnamon powder

1 tablespoon stevia

Directions:

Arrange apple slices in your air fryer's basket, add stevia and cinnamon, toss and cook at 390 degrees F for 10 minutes turning them halfway.

Transfer to a bowl and serve as a snack.

Enjoy!

Nutrition: calories 90, fat 0, fiber 4, carbs 12, protein 4

8. Potato Chips

Preparation Time: 30 minutes

Cooking time: 30 minutes

Servings: 4

Ingredients:

4 potatoes, scrubbed, peeled and cut into thin strips

A pinch of sea salt

1 tablespoon olive oil

2 teaspoons rosemary, chopped

Directions:

In a bowl, mix potato chips with salt and oil, toss to coat, place them in your air fryer's basket and cook at 330 degrees F for 30 minutes.

Divide them into bowls, sprinkle rosemary all over and serve as a snack.

Enjoy!

Nutrition: calories 200, fat 4, fiber 4, carbs 14, protein 5

9. Easy Zucchini Chips

Preparation Time: 10 minutes

Cooking time: 30 minutes

Servings: 6

Ingredients:

3 zucchinis, thinly sliced

Salt and black pepper to the taste

2 tablespoons olive oil

2 tablespoons balsamic vinegar

Directions:

In a bowl, mix oil with vinegar, salt and pepper and whisk well.

Add zucchini slices, toss to coat well, introduce in your air fryer and cook at 350 degrees F for 30 minutes.

Divide zucchini chips into bowls and serve them cold as a snack.

Enjoy!

Nutrition: calories 100, fat 3, fiber 2, carbs 6, protein 7

10. Beets Chips

Preparation Time: 10 minutes

Cooking time: 20 minutes

Servings: 4

Ingredients:

Cooking spray

4 medium beets, peeled and cut into very thin slices

Salt and black pepper to the taste

1 tablespoon chives, chopped

Directions:

Arrange beets chips in your air fryer's basket, grease with cooking spray, season with salt and black pepper, cook them at 350 degrees F for 20 minutes, flipping them halfway, transfer to bowls and serve with chives sprinkled on top as a snack

Enjoy!

Nutrition: calories 80, fat 1, fiber 2, carbs 6, protein 1

11. Avocado Chips

Preparation Time: 10 minutes

Cooking time: 10 minutes

Servings: 3

Ingredients:

1 avocado, pitted, peeled and sliced

Salt and black pepper to the taste

½ cup vegan breadcrumbs

A drizzle of olive oil

Directions:

In a bowl, mix breadcrumbs with salt and pepper and stir.

Brush avocado slices with the oil, coat them in breadcrumbs, place them in your air fryer's basket and cook at 390 degrees F for 10 minutes, shaking halfway.

Divide into bowls and serve them as a snack

Enjoy!

Nutrition: calories 180, fat 11, fiber 3, carbs 7, protein 4

12. Veggie Sticks

Preparation Time: 10 minutes

Cooking time: 30 minutes

Servings: 4

Ingredients:

4 parsnips, cut into thin sticks

2 sweet potatoes, cut into sticks

4 carrots, cut into sticks

Salt and black pepper to the taste

2 tablespoons rosemary, chopped

2 tablespoons olive oil

A pinch of garlic powder

Directions:

Put parsnips, sweet potatoes and carrots in a bowl, add oil, garlic powder, salt, pepper and rosemary and toss to coat.

Put sweet potatoes in your preheated air fryer, cook them for 10 minutes at 350 degrees F and transfer them to a platter.

Add parsnips to your air fryer, cook for 5 minutes and transfer over potato fries.

Add carrots, cook for 15 minutes at 350 degrees F, also transfer to the platter.

Serve as a snack.

Enjoy!

Nutrition: calories 140, fat 0, fiber 2, carbs 7, protein 4

13. Polenta Biscuits

Preparation Time: 10 minutes

Cooking time: 25 minutes

Servings: 4

Ingredients:

18 ounces cooked polenta roll, cold

1 tablespoon olive oil

Directions:

Cut polenta in medium slices and brush them with the olive oil.

Place polenta biscuits into your air fryer and cook at 400 degrees F for 25 minutes, flipping them after 10 minutes.

Serve biscuits as a snack.

Nutrition: calories 120, fat 0, fiber 3, carbs 7, protein 3

14. Potato And Beans Dip

Preparation Time: 10 minutes

Cooking time: 10 minutes

Servings: 10

Ingredients:

19 ounces canned garbanzo beans, drained

1 cup sweet potatoes, peeled and chopped

¼ cup sesame paste

2 tablespoons lemon juice

1 tablespoon olive oil

5 garlic cloves, minced

½ teaspoon cumin, ground

2 tablespoons water

Salt and white pepper to the taste

Directions:

Put potatoes in your air fryer's basket, cook them at 360 degrees F for 10 minutes, cool them down, peel, put them in your food processor and pulse well.

Add sesame paste, garlic, beans, lemon juice, cumin, water, oil, salt and pepper, pulse again, divide into bowls and serve cold.

Enjoy!

Nutrition: calories 170, fat 3, fiber 10, carbs 12, protein 11

15. Squash Party Muffins

Preparation Time: 10 minutes

Cooking time: 26 minutes

Servings: 6

Ingredients:

1 spaghetti squash, peeled and halved

2 tablespoons avocado mayonnaise

1 cup cashew cheese, shredded

1 and ½ cups vegan breadcrumbs

1 teaspoon parsley, dried

1 garlic clove, minced

Salt and black pepper to the taste

Cooking spray

Directions:

Put squash halves in your air fryer, cook at 350 degrees F for 16 minutes, leave aside to cool down, scrape flesh into a bowl, add salt, pepper, parsley, breadcrumbs, mayo and cashew cheese and stir well.

Spray a muffin tray that fits your air fryer with cooking spray and divide squash mix in each cup, introduce in the fryer and cook at 360 degrees F for 10 minutes.

Arrange muffins on a platter and serve as a snack.

Enjoy!

Nutrition: calories 120, fat 2, fiber 3, carbs 7, protein 4

16. Cauliflower Crackers

Preparation Time: 10 minutes

Cooking time: 25 minutes

Servings: 12

Ingredients:

1 big cauliflower head, florets separated and riced

½ cup cashew cheese, shredded

1 tablespoon flax meal mixed with 1 tablespoon water

1 teaspoon Italian seasoning

Salt and black pepper to the taste

Directions:

Spread cauliflower rice on a lined baking sheet that fits your air fryer, introduce in the fryer and cook at 360 degrees F for 10 minutes.

Transfer cauliflower to a bowl, add salt, pepper, cashew cheese, flax meal and Italian seasoning, stir really well, spread this into a rectangle pan that fits your air fryer, press well, introduce in the fryer and cook at 360 degrees F for 15 minutes more.

Cut into medium crackers and serve as a snack.

Enjoy!

Nutrition: calories 120, fat 1, fiber 2, carbs 7, protein 3

17. Basil Crackers

Preparation Time: 10 minutes

Cooking time: 17 minutes

Servings: 6

Ingredients:

½ teaspoon baking powder

Salt and black pepper to the taste

1 and ¼ cups whole wheat flour

¼ teaspoon basil, dried

1 garlic clove, minced

2 tablespoons vegan basil pesto

2 tablespoons olive oil

Directions:

In a bowl, mix flour with salt, pepper, baking powder, garlic, cayenne, basil, pesto and oil, stir until you obtain a dough, spread this on a lined baking sheet that fits your air fryer, introduce in the fryer at 325 degrees F and bake for 17 minutes.

Leave aside to cool down, cut crackers and serve them as a snack.

Enjoy!

Nutrition: calories 170, fat 20, fiber 1, carbs 6, protein 7

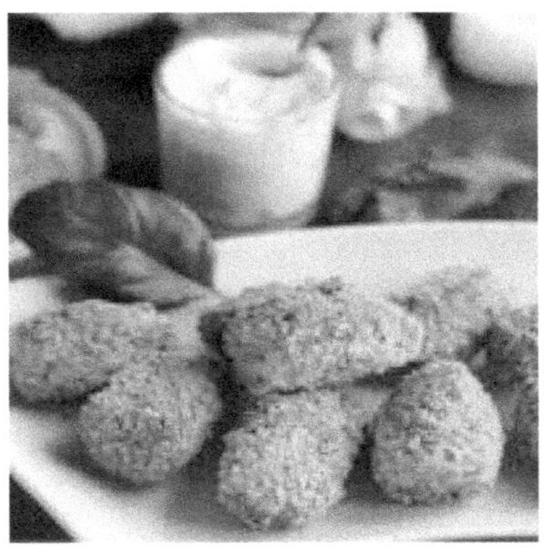

18. Banana Chips

Preparation Time: 10 minutes

Cooking Time: 10 minutes

Servings: 4

Ingredients

4 bananas, peeled and sliced in thin pieces

A drizzle of olive oil

A pinch of black pepper

Preparation

Put banana slices in your Air Fryer, drizzle the oil, season with pepper, toss to coat gently and cook at 360 ° for 10 minutes.

Serve as a snack.

Nutrition:

Calories 100, Fat 7g, Fiber 1g, Carbs 20g, Protein 1g

19. Tortilla Chips

Preparation Time: 10 minutes

Cooking Time: 4 minutes

Servings: 4

Ingredients

8 corn tortillas, each cut into triangles

Salt and black pepper to the taste

1 tablespoon olive oil

Directions:

Brush tortilla chips with the oil, place them in your Air Fryer's basket and cook for 4 minutes at 400 ° F

Serve them with salt and pepper sprinkled all over.

Nutrition:

Calories 53, Fat 1g, Fiber 1.5g, Carbs 10g, Protein 2g

20. Chickpeas Snack

Preparation Time: 10 minutes

Cooking Time: 20 minutes

Servings: 4

Ingredients

15 ounces canned chickpeas, drained

½ teaspoon cumin, ground

1 tablespoon olive oil

1 teaspoon smoked paprika

Salt and black pepper to the taste

Directions:

In a bowl, mix chickpeas with oil, cumin, paprika, salt and pepper, toss to coat, place them in the friar's basket, cook at 390 ° F for 10 minutes and transfer to a bowl.

Serve as a snack

Nutrition:

Calories 140, Fat 1g, Fiber 6g, Carbs 20g, Protein 6g

21. Apple Chips

Preparation Time: 10 minutes

Cooking Time: 15 minutes

Servings: 2

Ingredients

1 apple, cored and thinly sliced

½ teaspoon cinnamon powder

1 tablespoon stevia

Directions:

Arrange apple slices in your Air Fryer's basket, add stevia and cinnamon, toss and cook at 390 ° F for 10 minutes turning them halfway.

Transfer to a bowl and serve as a snack.

Nutrition:

Calories 90, Fat 0g, Fiber 4g, Carbs 12g, Protein 4g

22. Potato Chips

Preparation Time: 30 minutes

Cooking Time: 30 minutes

Servings: 4

Ingredients

4 potatoes, scrubbed, peeled and cut into thin strips

A pinch of sea salt

1 tablespoon olive oil

2 teaspoons rosemary, chopped

Preparation

In a bowl, mix potato chips with salt and oil, toss to coat, place them in your Air Fryer's basket and cook at 330 ° F for 30 minutes.

Divide them into bowls, sprinkle rosemary all over and serve as a snack.

Nutrition:

Calories 200, Fat 4g, Fiber 4g, Carbs 14g, Protein 5g

23. Easy Zucchini Chips

Preparation Time: 10 minutes

Cooking Time: 30 minutes

Servings: 6

Ingredients

3 zucchinis, thinly sliced

Salt and black pepper to the taste

2 tablespoons olive oil

2 tablespoons balsamic vinegar

Directions:

In a bowl, mix oil with vinegar, salt and pepper and whisk well.

Add zucchini slices, toss to coat well, introduce in your Air Fryer and cook at 350 ° F for 30 minutes.

Divide zucchini chips into bowls and serve them cold as a snack.

Nutrition:

Calories 100, Fat 3g, Fiber 2g, Carbs 6g, Protein 7g

24. Beets Chips

Preparation Time: 10 minutes

Cooking Time: 20 minutes

Servings: 4

Ingredients

Cooking spray

4 medium beets, peeled and cut into very thin slices

Salt and black pepper to the taste

1 tablespoon chives, chopped

Preparation

Arrange beets chips in your Air Fryer's basket, grease with cooking spray, season with salt and black pepper, cook them at 350 ° F for 20 minutes, flipping them halfway, transfer to bowls and serve with chives sprinkled on top as a snack.

Nutrition:

Calories 80, Fat 1g, Fiber 2g, Carbs 6g, Protein 1g

25. Avocado Chips

Preparation Time: 10 minutes

Cooking Time: 10 minutes

Servings: 3

Ingredients

1 avocado, pitted, peeled and sliced

Salt and black pepper to the taste

½ cup vegan breadcrumbs

A drizzle of olive oil

Directions:

In a bowl, mix breadcrumbs with salt and pepper and stir.

Brush avocado slices with the oil, coat them in breadcrumbs, place them in your Air Fryer's basket and cook at 390 ° F for 10 minutes, shaking halfway.

Divide into bowls and serve them as a snack

Nutrition:

Calories 180, Fat 11g, Fiber 3g, Carbs 7g, Protein 4g

26. Veggie Sticks

Preparation Time: 10 minutes

Cooking Time: 30 minutes

Servings: 4

Ingredients

4 parsnips, cut into thin sticks

2 sweet potatoes, cut into sticks

4 carrots, cut into sticks

Salt and black pepper to the taste

2 tablespoons rosemary, chopped

2 tablespoons olive oil

A pinch of garlic powder

Directions:

Put parsnips, sweet potatoes and carrots in a bowl, add oil, garlic powder, salt, pepper and rosemary and toss to coat.

Put sweet potatoes in your preheated Air Fryer, cook them for 10 minutes at 350 ° F and transfer them to a platter.

Add parsnips to your Air Fryer, cook for 5 minutes and transfer over potato fries.

Add carrots, cook for 15 minutes at 350 ° F, also transfer to the platter.

Serve as a snack.

Nutrition:

Calories 140, Fat 0g, Fiber 2g, Carbs 7g, Protein 4g

27. Polenta Biscuits

Preparation Time: 10 minutes

Cooking Time: 25 minutes

Servings: 4

Ingredients

18 ounces cooked polenta roll, cold

1 tablespoon olive oil

Preparation

Cut polenta in medium slices and brush them with the olive oil.

Place polenta biscuits into your Air Fryer and cook at 400 ° F for 25 minutes, flipping them after 10 minutes.

Serve biscuits as a snack.

Nutrition:

Calories 120, Fat 0g, Fiber 3g, Carbs 7g, Protein 3g

28. Cauliflower Crackers

Preparation Time: 10 minutes

Cooking Time: 25 minutes

Servings: 12

Ingredients

1 big cauliflower head, florets separated and riced

½ cup cashew cheese, shredded

1 tablespoon flax meal mixed with 1 tablespoon water

1 teaspoon Italian seasoning

Salt and black pepper to the taste

Preparation

Spread cauliflower rice on a lined baking sheet that fits your Air Fryer, introduce in the fryer and cook at 360 ° F for 10 minutes.

Transfer cauliflower to a bowl, add salt, pepper, cashew cheese, flax meal and Italian seasoning, stir really well, spread this into a rectangle pan that fits your Air Fryer, press well, introduce in the fryer and cook at 360 ° F for 15 minutes more.

Cut into medium crackers and serve as a snack.

Nutrition:

Calories 120, Fat 1g, Fiber 2g, Carbs 7g, Protein 3g

29. Basil Crackers

Preparation Time: 10 minutes

Cooking Time: 17 minutes

Servings: 6

Ingredients

½ teaspoon baking powder

Salt and black pepper to the taste

1¼ cups whole wheat flour

¼ teaspoon basil, dried

1 garlic clove, minced

2 tablespoons vegan basil pesto

2 tablespoons olive oil

Preparation

In a bowl, mix flour with salt, pepper, baking powder, garlic, cayenne, basil, pesto and oil, stir until you obtain a dough, spread this on a lined baking sheet that fits your Air Fryer, introduce in the fryer at 325 ° F and bake for 17 minutes.

Leave aside to cool down, cut crackers and serve them as a snack.

Nutrition:

Calories 170, Fat 20g, Fiber 1g, Carbs 6g, Protein 7g

30. Kale Crackers

Preparation Time: 10 minutes

Cooking Time: 20 minutes

Servings: 6

Ingredients

2 cups flaxseed, ground

2 cups flaxseed, soaked overnight and drained

4 bunches kale, chopped

1 bunch basil, chopped

4 garlic cloves, minced

1/3 cup olive oil

Preparation

In your food processor mix ground flaxseed with kale, basil and garlic and blend well.

Add oil and soaked flaxseed, blend again, spread in your Air Fryer's pan, cut into medium crackers and cook them at 380 ° F for 20 minutes.

Divide into bowls and serve as a snack.

Nutrition:

Calories 173, Fat 1g, Fiber 2g, Carbs 8g, Protein 4g

31. Squash Pate

Preparation Time: 10 minutes

Cooking Time: 25 minutes

Servings: 4

Ingredients

2 cups butternut squash, peeled and cubed

3 tablespoons coconut milk

A pinch of rosemary, dried

A pinch of sage, dried

A pinch of salt and black pepper

Preparation

In your Air Fryer's pan, mix squash, coconut milk, sage, rosemary, salt and pepper, toss, introduce in your Air Fryer and cook at 375 ° F for 25 minutes.

Blend using an immersion blender, divide into bowls and serve cold.

Nutrition:

Calories 182, Fat 5g, Fiber 7g, Carbs 12g, Protein 5g

32. Eggplant Appetizer Salad

Preparation Time: 10 minutes

Cooking Time: 20 minutes

Servings: 4

Ingredients

1½ cups tomatoes, chopped

3 cups eggplant, cubed

6 ounces black olives, pitted and sliced

2 teaspoons balsamic vinegar

1 tablespoon oregano, chopped

Salt and black pepper to the taste

Preparation

In a pan that fits your Air Fryer, mix tomatoes with eggplant, olives, vinegar, oregano, salt and pepper, toss, introduce in your fryer and cook at 370 ° F for 20 minutes.

Divide between small appetizer plates and serve as an appetizer.

Nutrition:

Calories 170, Fat 6g, Fiber 5g, Carbs 9g, Protein 2g

33. Vegan Veggie Dip

Preparation Time: 10 minutes

Cooking Time: 25 minutes

Servings: 4

Ingredients

1 cup carrots, sliced

1½ cups cauliflower florets

1/3 cup cashews

½ cup turnips, chopped

2½ cups water

1 cup almond milk

1 teaspoon garlic powder

¼ cup nutritional yeast

¼ teaspoon smoked paprika

¼ teaspoon mustard powder

A pinch of salt

Preparation

In a pan that fits your Air Fryer, mix carrots with cauliflower, cashews, turnips and water, stir, put in your Air Fryer and cook at 365 ° F for 25 minutes.

Transfer to a blender, add almond milk, garlic powder, yeast, paprika, mustard powder and salt, blend well and serve.

Nutrition:

Calories 261, Fat 7g, Fiber 4g, Carbs 14g, Protein 3g

34. Chickpeas Dip

Preparation Time: 10 minutes

Cooking Time: 20 minutes

Servings: 10

Ingredients

1 cup canned chickpeas, drained and some of the liquid reserved

2 tablespoons olive oil

1 tablespoon sesame paste

A pinch of salt and black pepper

1 garlic clove, minced

1 tablespoon lemon juice

Preparation

In a pan that fits your Air Fryer mix chickpeas with salt, pepper, lemon juice and oil, stir, transfer to your Air Fryer and cook at 365 ° F for 20 minutes.

Transfer chickpeas to a blender, add sesame paste, reserved liquid and garlic, blend well, divide into bowls and serve as a dip

Nutrition:

Calories 241, Fat 6g, Fiber 7g, Carbs 8g, Protein 4g

35. Spinach Spread

Preparation Time: 10 minutes

Cooking Time: 10 minutes

Servings: 4

Ingredients

½ cup coconut cream

¾ cup coconut yogurt

10 ounces spinach

8 ounces water chestnuts, chopped

1 garlic clove, minced

Preparation

In a pan that fits your Air Fryer, mix coconut cream with spinach, coconut yogurt, chestnuts and garlic, stir, transfer to your Air Fryer, cook at 365 ° F for 10 minutes, blend using an immersion blender, divide into bowls and serve as an appetizer.

Nutrition:

Calories 201, Fat 5g, Fiber 7g, Carbs 12g, Protein 5g

36. Avocado Fries

Servings: 4

Ingredients

Aquafaba from 1 15-ounce white beans or garbanzo beans

1 Haas avocado, peeled, pitted and sliced

1/2 teaspoon salt

1/2 cup panko breadcrumbs

Directions

In a bowl, mix together the panko breadcrumbs and the salt and then place the aquafaba in another bowl.

Dip the avocado slices into the aquafaba and then dip them into the panko. Try to get an even coating. Proceed to place the slices in your air fryer basket in a single layer. They should not overlap.

Air fry the avocado fries for 10 minutes at 390 degrees F. Be sure to shake the air fryer after 5 minutes.

Serve immediately with your dipping sauce of choice.

Nutrition: Calories 239, Carb 32.97g, Fat 7.88g, Protein 11.67g

37. Air Fried Tofu

Servings: 4

Ingredients

1 tablespoon potato starch or cornstarch

2 teaspoons toasted sesame oil

1 teaspoon seasoned rice vinegar

2 tablespoons soy sauce

1 block firm tofu, pressed and cut into 1-inch cubes

Directions

In a bowl, mix together the tofu, vinegar, oil and soy sauce and allow the mixture to marinate for about 15-30 minutes.

Add the cornstarch and toss then pour the mixture in your air fryer basket. Proceed to cook for 20 minutes at 370. Be sure to shake the air fryer after 10 minutes.

Serve and enjoy.

Nutrition: Calories 168, Carbs 7.28g, Fat 10.76g, Protein 13.35g

38. Pineapple In Air Fryer

Servings: 8

Ingredients

8 slices pineapple

Salt to taste

Directions

Carefully peel the pineapple and slice it into 8 slices. Sprinkle the pieces with some salt and then cook them at 160 degrees C for 10 minutes.

Serve and enjoy.

Nutrition: Calories 28, Carbs 15.0g, Fat 0.04g, Protein 0.2g

39. Air Fryer Sweet Potato

Servings: 3

Ingredients

1-2 teaspoons kosher salt

1 tablespoon olive oil

3 sweet potato

Directions

Carefully wash the sweet potatoes and then use a fork to poke air holes into them. Season the sweet potatoes with salt and olive oil. Ensure you rub the seasoning evenly.

Arrange the potatoes inside your air fryer basket and then cook for 35-40 minutes at 392 degrees F. The potatoes should be fork tender once don't.

Serve with your favorite toppings.

Nutrition: Calories 153, Carbs 26.16g, Fats 4.57g, Proteins 2.04g

40. Air Fryer Carrot Chips

Servings: 2

Ingredients

Toppings: rosemary, thyme and paprika or cardamon, nutmeg and cinnamon

4 carrots, fresh or frozen, rainbow or orange

Carrot dip:

8 oz. sour cream, vegan

Salt and pepper to taste

Lemon to taste

Dill

Onion powder

1 teaspoon garlic powder

Directions

Preheat your air fryer to 400 degrees F.

Slice the carrots with a knife. The pieces should not be too thick. If you are using frozen carrots, first thaw them under warm water.

Sprinkle the carrot slices with salt to taste and then arrange them inside your air fryer basket. Cook for 12 minutes, shaking twice.

Serve with dip.

Nutrition: Calories 150, Fat 9.0g, Carbs 15.0g, Protein 2.0g

41. Crispy Air Fryer Tofu (Vegan, Gluten-Free)

Servings: 2

Ingredients

1 teaspoon water

1 teaspoon sesame oil

2 tablespoons soy sauce or tamari, to make it gluten-free

1/2 teaspoon garlic powder

1 tablespoon brown rice flour

2 tablespoons nutritional yeast

1 8-ounce package of firm tofu, rinsed and cubed

Directions

In a small bowl, combine the dry ingredients before adding the wet ingredients and stirring. Pour the mixture over the tofu and let it marinate for 30 minutes.

Sprinkle 1 tablespoon of brown rice flour and then mix it up just before placing the tofu in the air fryer.

Cook for 18 minutes at 350 degrees F.

Nutrition: Calories 278, Carbs 10g, Fat 12g, Protein 34g

42. Faux-Fried Pickle Chips

Servings: 2 (12 pickle chips)

Ingredients

Optional dip: ketchup, light Thousand Island dressing

1/4 cup fat-free liquid egg substitute

24 hamburger dill pickle chips

Dash each salt and black pepper

Dash cayenne pepper

1/4 teaspoon onion powder

1/4 teaspoon garlic powder

1/3 cup whole-wheat panko breadcrumbs

Directions

In a bowl, mix together the seasonings and breadcrumbs.

Carefully blot the pickle chips dry and then put them in a bowl. Coat the chips with the egg substitute and then shake each piece to remove excess egg substitute.

Coat the pickles with the seasoned breadcrumbs and then arrange them in your air fryer basket and top with remaining crumbs.

Cook for 3-4 minutes at 392 degrees. They should be golden brown.

Serve.

Nutrition: Calories 58, Fat 0.5g, Carbs 11.5g, Protein 2.5g

43. Air Fryer Sweet Potato Fries

Servings: 2

Ingredients

Fresh black pepper, to taste

1/4 teaspoon sweet paprika

1/2 teaspoon garlic powder

1/2 teaspoon kosher salt

2 teaspoons olive oil

2 medium peeled sweet potatoes (12 oz total)

Directions

Preheat your air fryer to 400 degrees F (8 minutes).

Spray the basket with some oil.

Slice the potatoes into 1/4-inch thick fries and then toss the slices with oil, paprika, black pepper, garlic powder and salt.

Cook the fries in 2-3 batches for 8 minutes. Turn halfway.

Serve and enjoy.

Nutrition: Calories 221, Fat 5g, Carbs 42g, Protein 3g

44. Crispy Air Fried Black-Eyed Peas

Servings: 6

Ingredients

1/8 teaspoon smoked salt

1/8 teaspoon black pepper

1/8 teaspoon chipotle chili sauce

1/4 teaspoon salt, optional

1/2 teaspoon chili powder

1 15-ounce can black-eyed peas (or 12/3 cups firmly cooked, not mushy)

Directions

Drain the liquid from the black-eyed peas then rinse off with running water and allow them to drain in a colander for a few minutes. Place the peas on a plate. Discard mushy peas.

In a bowl, mix together the seasoning ingredients and then proceed to sprinkle the mixture over the peas. Stir gently to coat the peas.

Preheat the air fryer to 350-360 degrees F and then air fry the peas for 10 minutes. Make sure you shake the air fryer after 5 minutes.

Remove and allow to cook and then serve while warm.

Nutrition: Calories 82, Fat 0.28g, Carbs 14.71g, Protein 2.48g

45. Roasted Garlic

Servings: 1

Ingredients

Drizzle extra virgin olive oil

1 medium sized head garlic

Directions

Peel the garlic but leave each clove covered and then cut off 1/4 inch off the heads to expose the cloves underneath.

Proceed to drizzle the oil into the parts that are exposed and then wrap the garlic in a piece of aluminum foil. Place the foil into your air fryer.

Cook for 20 minutes at 400 degrees. Check the doneness and increase cooking time if needed.

Allow to cool and then squeeze each clove so that it pops from the skin.

Serve with warmed bread. You can use the roasted garlic as a pizza topping if you wish.

Nutrition: Calories 4.5, Fat 0.1g, Carbs 1.0g, Protein 0.2g

46. Potato Chip Crusted Fried Green Tomatoes

Servings: 2

Ingredients

Spritz of oil (if using panko breadcrumbs)

1 medium-sized green tomato, thinly sliced

Pinch of salt and pepper

1/2 teaspoon granulated onion

1/2 teaspoon dried oregano

1/2 teaspoon dried basil

1/4 cup vegan mayonnaise

3 tablespoons cornstarch

1/2 cup potato chip crumbs (from 3 big handfuls potato chips) or panko breadcrumbs

Directions

Crumble the potato chips in a food processor.

Place vegan mayonnaise on a plate and then place the potato chips crumbs on another plate and put the cornstarch on a third plate.

Combine the crumbs, salt, pepper, granulated onion, dried oregano and basil.

Use a clean towel to blot the green tomato slices and then proceed to dip each tomato slice into the cornstarch. Cover the slices completely and then tap the tomato slices to remove excess cornstarch. Next, dip the slices in the vegan mayonnaise and lastly the crumb mixture.

Arrange the slices in the air fryer in an even layer. Spritz with oil (if you're using breadcrumbs) and then cook for 7 minutes at 400 degrees F. Do not shake or flip the air fryer. If you're using breadcrumbs, flip after 5-7 minutes, spritz more oil and cook for 2 more minutes.

Season with salt and serve.

Nutrition: Calories 312, Fat 18.0g, Carbs 29.9g, Protein 6.7g

47. Air Fried Potato Peels

Servings: 1

Ingredients

Optional toppings: ketchup, green onions, nondairy cream cheese, seitan bacon, sautéed minced garlic

Pinch of salt

Spritz of oil

Peels from 2 pounds of Russet potatoes (about 4 medium-sized potatoes)

Directions

Place the potato peels inside your air fryer basket and then spritz them with oil. Add a pinch of salt but do not over salt them.

Cook for 6-8 minutes at 400 degrees F. Make sure you shake the basket halfway through and spritz the peels with some more oil. The peels should be brown and crisp.

Serve immediately with your desired toppings.

Nutrition: Calories 110, Fat 0.1g, Carbs 11.0g, Protein 4.0g

48. Beetroot Chips

Servings: 1

Ingredients

Pepper, optional

Salt to taste

1 tablespoon oil

2 medium sized beetroots

Directions

Wash the beetroots and then peel the skin. Carefully slice the beetroot into slices and then place them on a paper and cover with another paper for 19 minutes. This will get rid of excess moisture.

Season with salt and then preheat the air fryer to 150 degrees C. This should take 4 minutes. Place the beetroot thins inside the air fryer and cook for 15 minutes. Shake every 5 minutes. Once the chips are slightly crisp, allow them to cool before cooking for a few more minutes.

Season with salt and ground pepper if you wish.

Nutrition: Calories 35, Fat 0.1g, Carbs 7.8g, Protein 1.3g

49. Banana Chips

Servings: 2

Ingredients

Little oil for the air fryer

Salt

Black pepper

4 raw bananas

Directions

Peel and slice the bananas into thin chips and then mix the chips with some oil.

Place the slices into the air fryer and cook at 180 degrees C for 10 minutes.

Serve with salt and pepper.

Nutrition: Calories 147.1, Fat 9.5g, Carbs 16.6g, Protein 0.7g

50. Air Fryer Brussels Sprouts

Servings: 2

Ingredients

1/4 teaspoon sea salt

1 tablespoon balsamic vinegar

1 tablespoon olive oil or maple syrup for oil-free option

2 cups halved Brussels sprouts, sliced lengthwise

Directions

In a bowl, mix together the Brussels sprouts, salt, oil and vinegar.

Cook for 8-10 minutes at 400 degrees F. Check progress at the 5 minutes mark. The sprouts should be browned and crispy.

Serve.

Nutrition: Calories 72, Carbs 9.24g, Fat 3.26g, Proteins 3.04g

51. Air Fryer Apple Chips

Servings: 1

Ingredients

1 teaspoon nutmeg

1/4 teaspoon cinnamon

1 medium apple

Directions

Preheat your air fryer to 375 degrees F.

Thinly slice the apple and then mix together with nutmeg and cinnamon.

Place the seasoned apple slices inside your air fryer basket and then bake for 8 minutes. Ensure you flip halfway.

Remove and serve.

Nutrition: Calories 108, Carbs 26.78g, Fats 1.12g, Proteins 0.63g

52. Air Fried Asparagus

Servings: 2

Ingredients

Black pepper

Himalayan salt

Avocado oil or olive oil

1/2 bunch of asparagus, with bottom 2 inches trimmed off

Directions

Arrange the asparagus in the air fryer and then spritz lightly with oil. Add salt and black pepper and then cook for 10 minutes at 400.

Serve immediately.

Nutrition: Calories 25.0, Fat 0.0g, Carbs 4.0g, Protein 2.0g

53. Air Fried Kale Chips

Servings: 2

Ingredients

1/4 teaspoon Himalayan salt

3 tablespoons nutritional yeast

Avocado oil or olive oil in a spritzer

1 bunch kale

Directions

Rinse the kale and then dry it with paper towels. Tear the leaves into 3-inch pieces.

Place the pieces in the bowl and spritz 10-12 times with oil. Add salt and nutritional yeast and mix it up using your hands. Massage the oil onto the leaves.

Cook for 5 minutes at 350 degrees. Cook in batches to avoid overcrowding.

Nutrition: Calories 227, Fat 15.29g, Carbs 17.02g, Protein 9.89g

54. Air Fryer Tater Tots

Servings: 3

Ingredients

1 tablespoon garlic salt

1 teaspoon garlic powder

1 tablespoon chives, minced

2 tablespoons cornstarch

2 tablespoons dehydrated chopped onion or 1/2 cup freshly minced

3 large Russet potatoes, cleaned and peeled

Directions

Preheat the air fryer to 400 degrees F.

In a bowl, add 2 tablespoons of dehydrated onions and 2 tablespoons of hot water and then set aside.

Peel and wash the potatoes and then grate them. Cover them with cold water, strain and rinse. Make sure you squeeze out excess water.

Place the grated potatoes in a bowl and mix together with cornstarch. Cook for 20 minutes in the air fryer. Alternatively, you can bake in an oven.

Allow the potatoes to cool and then mix them with chives, garlic salt, onions and garlic powder.

Form the potatoes into a tight ball. Each ball should be 1-2 tablespoons of potato mixture.

Air fry the potato balls for 20 minutes at 350 degrees. Shake occasionally.

Remove and serve.

Nutrition: Calories 350, Fat 0.4g, Carbs 80.44g, Protein 9.14g

55. Garlicky Air Fryer Roasted Almonds

Servings: 8

Ingredients

2 cups raw almonds

1/4 teaspoon pepper

1 teaspoon paprika

1 tablespoon garlic powder

Directions

In a bowl, mix together all the ingredients minus the almonds. Once a thick paste forms, add the almonds and coat them evenly.

Place the almonds in the air fryer and cook for 6-8 minutes at 320 degrees F. Shake the basket every 2 minutes.

Cool for 10-15 minutes and then serve. You can store them for 2-3 days at room temperature in an airtight container.

Nutrition: Calories 7, Fats 0.2g, Carbs 1.24g, Proteins 0.33g

56. Carrot Cake In A Mug

Servings: 1

Ingredients

2 teaspoons mild oil or applesauce or mashed banana for oil-free

1 tablespoon raisins or chopped dates

2 tablespoons grated carrot

2 tablespoons plus 2 teaspoons unsweetened nondairy milk

1 pinch salt

1 pinch allspice

1/8 teaspoon ground dried ginger

1/4 teaspoon ground cinnamon

1/4 teaspoon baking powder

1 tablespoon sweetener of choice

1/4 cup whole wheat parsley flour or your favorite blend

Directions

Carefully oil an oven-safe mug.

Add the flour, allspice, sugar, ginger, cinnamon, salt and baking powder and use a fork to mix well.

Add the milk, oil, raisins, carrot and walnuts and proceed to mix again. Cook for 15 minutes at 350 degrees F- Check to see if it is done. You can cook for 5 more minutes if needed.

Nutrition: Calories 117.7, Total Carbs 22.5g, Total Fat 2.8g, Protein 1.4g

57. Vegan Air Fryer Berry Cake

Servings: 4

Ingredients

2/3-3/4 cup mixed berries

1 teaspoon lemon peel

1 tablespoon vegetable oil

1 teaspoon white vinegar

3/4 cup soy milk

2/3 cup xylitol

1.5 cups whole meal self-rising flour

Directions

Use nonstick spray to spray a 6-inch cake pan.

Mix together the oil and xylitol.

Whisk the vinegar and soy milk and set aside to allow the mixture to curdle and then combine the two mixtures and stir in the oil, berries and lemon peel.

Add the flour and mix gently to form a batter.

Place the batter in the prepared pan and bake in the air fryer at 175 degrees C for 18-20 minutes.

Remove, cool and invert onto a serving plate.

Nutrition: Calories 350, Fat 10.0g, Carbs 58.0g, Protein 7.0g

58. Za'atar Spiced Air-Fried Kale Chips

Servings: 2

Ingredients

1/2-1 teaspoon sea salt

1-2 tablespoons za'atar seasoning

1 tablespoon olive oil

1 large bunch kale, de-stemmed, washed and spun - torn into bite size pieces

Directions

In a large mixing bowl, mix together the dried kale and olive oil and then gently massage the kale to coat well.

Add the seasonings and then mix well.

Cook in batches at 170 degrees C for 15-20 minutes per batch. Keep an eye on the chips to prevent burning.

Nutrition: Calories 200, Fat 14.0g, Carbs 9.0g, Protein 8.0g

59. Garlic And Herb Air Fryer Roasted Chickpeas

Servings: 4

Ingredients

Seal salt and black pepper to taste

1 tablespoon mixed herbs (oregano, thyme, rosemary)

2 teaspoons garlic powder

1 tablespoon nutritional yeast

1 tablespoon olive oil

2 cans of chickpeas

Directions

Drain the chickpeas and then rinse them and place them in a mixing bowl. Add the seasonings and olive oil and then stir to combine. The chickpeas should be well coated.

Divide into 2 batches and cook for 15-20 minutes at 200 degrees C. Stir halfway through.

Serve warm or store in an air-tight jar.

Nutrition: Calories 140, Fat 5.0g, Carbs 17.0g, Protein 6.0g

60. Crispy Fried Pickles

Servings: 14

Ingredients

1/4-1/2 cup vegan ranch dressing

Oil spray

Pinch of cayenne pepper

1/2 teaspoon paprika

6 tablespoons panko breadcrumbs

2 tablespoons cornstarch

2-3 tablespoons water

Pinch of salt

3 tablespoons datk beer (All German vegan beer)

1/8 teaspoon baking powder

1/4 cup all purpose flour

14 thickly cut dill pickle slices

Directions

Dry the pickle slices with a towel and set aside.

In a bowl, mix together the baking powder, all-purpose flour, 2 tablespoons of water, dark beer and a pinch of salt to get a waffle-like batter. You can add 1 more tablespoon of water if it is too thick.

In a plate, add the cornstarch. In another plate, add panko breadcrumbs, cayenne pepper, paprika and a pinch of salt.

Dip the pickles in the cornstarch and then the beer batter and lastly the panko mixture.

Arrange the pieces in the air fryer basket and spritz with spray oil. Air fry at 360 degrees for 8 minutes. Flip halfway and add a spritz of oil. You can cook for 1 more minute if needed.

Serve the pickles with vegan ranch dressing.

Nutrition: Calories 30, Fat 0.4g, Carbs 5.5g, Protein 1.3g

Next, we will discuss some tips, which will help you to use the air fryer effectively.

Chapter 4 Side Dishes

61. French Fries

Preparation Time: 40 minutes

Cooking Time: 30 minutes

Servings: 3

Ingredients:

2 potatoes, sliced into thick strips

1 bowl water

2 tablespoons olive oil

Salt and pepper to taste

¼ teaspoon paprika

1 tablespoon cornstarch

Cooking spray

Green onion, chopped

Method:

Soak potato strips in water for 30 minutes.

Drain and pat try.

Toss in olive oil.

Season with salt, pepper and paprika.

Cover with cornstarch.

Spray air fryer basket with oil.

Cook at 360 degrees F for 30 minutes shaking every 5 minutes.

Garnish with green onion.

Nutrition:

Calories 185

Total Fat 9 g

Saturated Fat 1 g

Cholesterol 0 mg

Sodium 297 mg

Total Carbohydrate 23 g

Dietary Fiber 2 g

Total Sugars 1 g

Protein 2 g

Potassium 482 mg

62. Crispy Zucchini Wedges

Preparation Time: 10 minutes

Cooking Time: 12 minutes

Servings: 6

Ingredients:

Cooking spray

½ cup all-purpose flour

2 vegan eggs

2 tablespoons water

1 ½ breadcrumbs

1 zucchini, sliced into wedges

½ tablespoon red-wine vinegar

2 tablespoons tomato paste

Salt and pepper to taste

Method:

Spray air fryer basket with oil.

Put the flour in a dish.

In another dish, combine vegan eggs and water.

In a third dish, put the breadcrumbs.

Dip each zucchini strip into the three dishes, first the flour, then the eggs and water, and lastly the breadcrumbs.

Cook in the air fryer at 360 degrees F for 12 minutes, shaking once.

Mix the rest of the ingredients in a bowl.

Serve zucchini fries with dipping sauce.

Nutrition:

Calories 235

Total Fat 12 g

Saturated Fat 1 g

Cholesterol 66 mg

Sodium 232 mg

Total Carbohydrate 26 g

Dietary Fiber 2 g

Total Sugars 2 g

Protein 6 g

Potassium 435 mg

63. Sweet Potato Chips

Preparation Time: 40 minutes

Cooking Time: 15 minutes

Servings: 4

Ingredients:

1 sweet potato, sliced into thin rounds

1 bowl water

1 tablespoon olive oil

Salt and pepper to taste

Cooking spray

Method:

Soak sweet potato slices in a bowl of water for 30 minutes.

Drain and then dry with paper towels.

Toss in oil and season with salt and pepper.

Spray air fryer basket with oil.

Cook sweet potato at 350 degrees F for 15 minutes, shaking every 5 minutes.

Nutrition:

Calories 62

Total Fat 4 g

Saturated Fat 1 g

Cholesterol 10 mg

Sodium 169 mg

Total Carbohydrate 14 g

Dietary Fiber 1 g

Total Sugars 1 g

Protein 0 g

Potassium 160 mg

64. Baked Potatoes With Broccoli & Cheese

Preparation Time: 10 minutes

Cooking Time: 30 minutes

Servings: 8

Ingredients:

4 potatoes

1 cup almond milk, divided

2 tablespoons all-purpose flour

½ cup vegan cheese, divided

1 cup broccoli, florets, chopped

Salt to taste

Chopped onion chives

Method:

Poke all sides of potatoes with a fork.

Microwave on high level for 5 minutes.

Flip and microwave for another 5 minutes.

In a saucepan over medium heat, heat ¾ cup of milk for 2 minutes, stirring frequently.

Add the remaining milk in a bowl and stir in the flour.

Add this mixture to the pan and bring to a boil.

Reduce heat

Reserve 2 tablespoons vegan cheese.

Add the rest of the cheese to the pan and stir until smooth.

Add the broccoli, salt and cayenne.

Cook for 1 minute and remove from heat.

Slice the potatoes and arrange on a single layer inside the air fryer.

Top with the broccoli mixture.

Add another layer of potatoes and broccoli mixture.

Sprinkle reserved cheese on top.

Cook at 350 degrees F for 5 minutes.

Garnish with chopped chives.

Nutrition:

Calories 137

Total Fat 3 g

Saturated Fat 2 g

Cholesterol 9 mg

Sodium 112 mg

Total Carbohydrate 148 g

Dietary Fiber 2 g

Total Sugars 3 g

Protein 5 g

Potassium 556 mg

65. Kale Chips

Preparation Time: 5 minutes

Cooking Time: 10 minutes

Servings: 2

Ingredients:

Cooking spray

6 cups kale leaves, torn

1 tablespoon olive oil

Salt to taste

1 ½ teaspoons low-sodium soy sauce

¼ teaspoon ground cumin

½ teaspoon white sesame seeds

Method:

Spray air fryer basket with oil.

Toss kale in oil, salt and soy sauce.

Cook at 375 degrees F for 10 minutes or until crispy. Shake every 3 minutes.

Sprinkle with cumin and sesame seeds before serving.

Nutrition:

Calories 140

Total Fat 9 g

Saturated Fat 1 g

Cholesterol 0 mg

Sodium 329 mg

Total Carbohydrate 13 g

Dietary Fiber 4 g

Total Sugars 3 g

Protein 4 g

Potassium 497 mg

66. Garlic Mushrooms

Preparation Time: 10 minutes

Cooking Time: 15 minutes

Servings: 2

Ingredients:

8 oz. mushrooms, rinsed, dried and sliced in half

1 tablespoon olive oil

½ teaspoon garlic powder

Salt and pepper to taste

1 teaspoon Worcestershire sauce

1 tablespoon parsley, chopped

Method:

Toss mushrooms in oil.

Season with garlic powder, salt, pepper and Worcestershire sauce.

Cook at 380 degrees F for 10 minutes, shaking halfway through.

Top with parsley before serving.

Nutrition:

Calories 90

Total Fat 7.4g

Saturated Fat 1g

Cholesterol 0mg

Sodium 35mg

Total Carbohydrate 4.9g

Dietary Fiber 1.3g

Total Sugars 2.6g

Protein 3.8g

Potassium 379mg

67. Rosemary Potatoes

Preparation Time: 15 minutes

Cooking Time: 15 minutes

Servings: 4

Ingredients:

4 potatoes, cubed

1 tablespoon oil

1 tablespoon garlic, minced

2 teaspoons dried rosemary, minced

Salt and pepper to taste

1 tablespoon lime juice

¼ cup parsley, chopped

Method:

Toss potato cubes in oil and season with garlic, rosemary, salt and pepper.

Put in the air fryer.

Cook at 400 degrees F for 15 minutes.

Stir in lime juice and top with parsley before serving.

Nutrition:

Calories 244

Total Fat 10.5g

Saturated Fat 2.1g

Cholesterol 0mg

Sodium 16mg

Total Carbohydrate 35g

Dietary Fiber 5.6g

Total Sugars 2.6g

Protein 3.9g

Potassium 905mg

68. Roasted Spicy Carrots

Preparation Time: 5 minutes

Cooking Time: 15 minutes

Servings: 4

Ingredients:

½ lb. carrots, sliced

½ tablespoon olive oil

Salt to taste

1/8 teaspoon garlic powder

¼ teaspoon chili powder

1 teaspoon ground cumin

Sesame seeds

Fresh cilantro

Method:

Preheat your air fryer at 390 degrees F for 5 minutes.

Cook the carrots at 390 degrees F for 10 minutes.

Transfer to a bowl.

Mix the oil, salt, garlic powder, chili powder and ground cumin.

Coat the carrots with the oil mixture.

Put the carrots back to the air fryer and cook for another 5 minutes.

Garnish with sesame seeds and cilantro.

Nutrition:

Calories 82

Total Fat 3.8g

Saturated Fat 0.5g

Cholesterol 0mg

Sodium 161mg

Total Carbohydrate 11.9g

Dietary Fiber 3g

Total Sugars 5.7g

Protein 1.2g

Potassium 390mg

69. Baked Artichoke Fries

Preparation Time: 10 minutes

Cooking Time: 10 minutes

Servings: 4

Ingredients:

14 oz. canned artichoke hearts, drained, rinsed and sliced into wedges

1 cup all-purpose flour

½ cup almond milk

½ teaspoon garlic powder

Salt and pepper to taste

1 ½ cup breadcrumbs

½ teaspoon paprika

Method:

Dry the artichoke hearts by pressing a paper towel on top.

In a bowl, mix the flour, milk, garlic powder, salt and pepper.

In a shallow dish, add the paprika and breadcrumbs.

Dip each artichoke wedge in the first bowl and then coat with the breadcrumb mixture.

Cook at 450 degrees for 10 minutes.

Serve fries with your choice of dipping sauce.

Nutrition:

Calories 391

Total Fat 9.8g

Saturated Fat 6.9g

Cholesterol 0mg

Sodium 395mg

Total Carbohydrate 65.5g

Dietary Fiber 8.8g

Total Sugars 4.7g

Protein 12.7g

Potassium 569mg

70. Baked Tofu Strips

Preparation Time: 30 minutes

Cooking Time: 40 minutes

Servings: 4

Ingredients:

2 tablespoons olive oil

½ teaspoon oregano

½ teaspoon basil

¼ teaspoon cayenne pepper

¼ teaspoon paprika

¼ teaspoon garlic powder

¼ teaspoon onion powder

Salt and pepper to taste

15 oz. tofu, drained

Method:

Combine all the ingredients except the tofu.

Mix well.

Slice tofu into strips and dry with paper towel.

Marinate in the mixture for 10 minutes.

Cook in the air fryer at 375 degrees F for 15 minutes, shaking halfway through.

Nutrition:

Calories 132

Total Fat 10 g

Saturated Fat 1 g

Cholesterol 0 mg

Sodium 40 mg

Total Carbohydrate 3 g

Dietary Fiber 0 g

Total Sugars 1 g

Protein 7 g

Potassium 213 mg

71. Avocado Fries

Preparation Time: 10 minutes

Cooking Time: 10 minutes

Servings: 4

Ingredients:

Salt to taste

½ cup panko breadcrumbs

1 cup aquafaba liquid

1 avocado, sliced into strips

Method:

Mix the salt and breadcrumbs in a bowl.

In another bowl, pour the aquafaba liquid.

Dip each avocado strip into the liquid and then dredge with breadcrumbs.

Air fry at 390 degrees F for 10 minutes, shaking halfway through.

Nutrition:

Calories 111

Total Fat 9.9g

Saturated Fat 2.1g

Cholesterol 0mg

Sodium 59mg

Total Carbohydrate 6.2g

Dietary Fiber 3.6g

Total Sugars 0.3g

Protein 1.2g

Potassium 244mg

72. Crispy Vegetables

Preparation Time: 15 minutes

Cooking Time: 8 minutes

Servings: 4

Ingredients:

1 cup rice flour

1 tablespoon nutritional yeast flakes

2 tablespoons vegan egg powder

2/3 cup cold water

1 cup breadcrumbs

Salt and pepper to taste

1 cup squash, sliced into strips

1 cup zucchini, sliced into strips

½ cup green beans

½ cup cauliflower, sliced into florets

Cooking spray

Method:

Set up three bowls.

One is for the rice flour, another for the egg powder, nutritional yeast and water, another for the breadcrumbs.

Dip each of the vegetable slices in the first, second and third bowls.

Spray the air fryer basket with oil.

Cook at 380 degrees F for 8 minutes or until crispy.

Nutrition:

Calories 272

Total Fat 2.2g

Saturated Fat 0.5g

Cholesterol 0mg

Sodium 208mg

Total Carbohydrate 54.8g

Dietary Fiber 3.9g

Total Sugars 2.7g

Protein 7.9g

Potassium 284mg

73. Flavored Beets

Preparation Time: 10 minutes

Cooking Time: 10 minutes

Servings: 4

Ingredients

1½ pounds beets, peeled and quartered

A drizzle of olive oil

2 teaspoons orange zest, grated

2 tablespoons cider vinegar

½ cup orange juice

2 tablespoons stevia

2 scallions, chopped

2 teaspoons mustard

Directions:

Rub beets with the oil and orange juice, place them in your Air Fryer's basket and cook at 350 ° F for 10 minutes.

Transfer beets to a bowl, add scallions, orange zest, stevia, mustard and vinegar, toss, divide between plates and serve as a side dish.

Nutrition:

Calories 121, Fat 2g, Fiber 3g, Carbs 11g, Protein 4g

74. Creamy Brussels Sprouts

Preparation Time: 4 minutes

Cooking Time: 10 minutes

Servings: 4

Ingredients

1 pound Brussels sprouts, trimmed

Salt and black pepper to the taste

1 tablespoon mustard

2 tablespoons coconut cream

2 tablespoons dill, chopped

Directions:

Put Brussels sprouts in your Air Fryer's basket and cook them at 350 ° F for 10 minutes.

In a bowl, mix cream with mustard, dill, salt and pepper and whisk.

Add Brussels sprouts, toss, divide between plates and serve as a side dish.

Nutrition:

Calories 162, Fat 8g, Fiber 8g, Carbs 14g, Protein 5g

75. Baby Carrots And Parsley

Preparation Time: 10 minutes

Cooking Time: 10 minutes

Servings: 4

Ingredients

2 cups baby carrots

Salt and black pepper to the taste

1 tablespoon parsley, chopped

½ tablespoon olive oil

Directions:

In a pan that fits your Air Fryer, mix baby carrots with oil, salt, pepper and parsley, toss, introduce in your Air Fryer and cook at 350 ° F for 10 minutes.

Divide between plates and serve as a side dish.

Nutrition:

Calories 100, Fat 2g, Fiber 3g, Carbs 7g, Protein 4g

76. Chili Fennel

Preparation Time: 10 minutes

Cooking Time: 8 minutes

Servings: 4

Ingredients

2 fennel bulbs, cut into quarters

3 tablespoons olive oil

Salt and black pepper to the taste

1 garlic clove, minced

1 red chili pepper, chopped

¾ cup veggie stock

Juice of ½ lemon

Preparation

Heat up a pan that fits your Air Fryer with the oil over medium-high heat, add garlic and chili pepper, stir and cook for 2 minutes.

Add fennel, salt, pepper, stock and lemon juice, toss to coat, introduce in your Air Fryer and cook at 350 ° F for 6 minutes.

Divide between plates and serve as a side dish.

Nutrition:

Calories 100, Fat 4g, Fiber 8g, Carbs 4g, Protein 4g

77. Collard Greens And Tomatoes

Preparation Time: 10 minutes

Cooking Time: 10 minutes

Servings: 4

Ingredients

1 pound collard greens

¼ cup cherry tomatoes, halved

1 tablespoon apple cider vinegar

2 tablespoons veggie stock

Salt and black pepper to the taste

Directions:

In a pan that fits your Air Fryer, combine tomatoes, collard greens, vinegar, stock, salt and pepper, stir, introduce in your Air Fryer and cook at 320 ° F for 10 minutes.

Divide between plates and serve as a side dish.

Nutrition:

Calories 150, Fat 3g, Fiber 1g, Carbs 5g, Protein 7g

78. Glazed Beets

Preparation Time: 10 minutes

Cooking Time: 50 minutes

Servings: 8

Ingredients

3 pounds beetroots, peeled and cut into medium chunks

4 tablespoons maple syrup

1 tablespoon olive oil

Directions:

Rub beets with the oil, add maple syrup, toss, introduce in your Air Fryer and cook at 350 ° F for 40 minutes.

Divide between plates and serve as a side dish.

Nutrition:

Calories 108, Fat 1g, Fiber 1.2g, Carbs 12g, Protein 1g

79. Paprika Broccoli

Preparation Time: 10 minutes

Cooking Time: 20 minutes

Servings: 4

Ingredients

1 broccoli head, florets separated

Juice of ½ lemon

1 tablespoon olive oil

2 teaspoons paprika

Salt and black pepper to the taste

3 garlic cloves, minced

1 tablespoon sesame seeds

Directions:

In a bowl, mix broccoli with lemon juice, oil, paprika, salt, pepper and garlic and toss to coat.

Transfer to your Air Fryer's basket, cook at 360 ° F for 15 minutes, sprinkle sesame seeds, cook for 5 minutes more, divide between plates and serve as a side dish.

Nutrition:

Calories 96, Fat 4g, Fiber 3g, Carbs 12g, Protein 5g

80. Easy Peppers Side Dish

Preparation Time: 10 minutes

Cooking Time: 25 minutes

Servings: 12

Ingredients

12 colored bell peppers, seedless and sliced

1 tablespoon olive oil

1 yellow onion, sliced

½ teaspoon smoked paprika

Salt and black pepper to the taste

Preparation

Put the oil in a pan that fits your Air Fryer, add bell peppers, paprika and onion, toss, introduce the pan in your Air Fryer and cook at 320 ° F for 25 minutes.

Season with salt and pepper to the taste, divide between plates and serve as a side dish.

Nutrition:

Calories 101, Fat 1g, Fiber 3g, Carbs 10g, Protein 2g

81. Cajun Onion Mix

Preparation Time: 2 hours

Cooking Time: 15 minutes

Servings: 4

Ingredients

2 big white onions, cut into medium chunks

Salt and black pepper to the taste

¼ cup coconut cream

A drizzle of olive oil

1½ teaspoon paprika

1 teaspoon garlic powder

½ teaspoon Cajun seasoning

Directions:

In a pan that fits your Air Fryer, combine onion chunks with salt, pepper, cream, oil, paprika, garlic powder and Cajun seasoning, toss, introduce the pan in your Air Fryer and cook at 360 ° F for 15 minutes.

Divide the onion mix between plates and serve as a side dish.

Nutrition:

Calories 200, Fat 2g, Fiber 2g, Carbs 8g, Protein 7g

82. Tomatoes And Basil Mix

Preparation Time: 10 minutes

Cooking Time: 14 minutes

Servings: 2

Ingredients

1 bunch basil, chopped

3 garlic clove, minced

A drizzle of olive oil

Salt and black pepper to the taste

2 cups cherry tomatoes, halved

Directions:

In a pan that fits your Air Fryer, combine tomatoes with garlic, salt, pepper, basil and oil, toss, introduce in your Air Fryer and cook at 320 ° F for 12 minutes.

Divide between plates and serve as a side dish.

Nutrition:

Calories 140, Fat 1g, Fiber 1g, Carbs 2g, Protein 10g

83. Green Beans Side Salad

Preparation Time: 10 minutes

Cooking Time: 15 minutes

Servings: 4

Ingredients

1-pint cherry tomatoes

1 pound green beans

2 tablespoons olive oil

Salt and black pepper to the taste

Preparation

In a bowl, mix cherry tomatoes with green beans, olive oil, salt and pepper, toss, and transfer to a pan that fits your Air Fryer and cook at 400 ° F for 15 minutes.

Divide between plates and serve as a side dish.

Nutrition:

Calories 142, Fat 6g, Fiber 5g, Carbs 8g, Protein 9g

84. Red Potatoes And Green Beans

Preparation Time: 10 minutes

Cooking Time: 15 minutes

Servings: 4

Ingredients

1 pound red potatoes, cut into wedges

1 pound green beans

2 garlic cloves, minced

2 tablespoons olive oil

Salt and black pepper to the taste

½ teaspoon oregano, dried

Directions:

In a pan that fits your Air Fryer, combine potatoes with green beans, garlic, oil, salt, pepper and oregano, toss, introduce in your Air Fryer and cook at 380 ° F for 15 minutes.

Divide between plates and serve as a side dish.

Nutrition:

Calories 201, Fat 6g, Fiber 4g, Carbs 8g, Protein 5g

85. White Mushrooms Mix

Preparation Time: 10 minutes

Cooking Time: 15 minutes

Servings: 2

Ingredients

Salt and black pepper to the taste

7 ounces snow peas

8 ounces white mushrooms, halved

1 yellow onion, cut into rings

2 tablespoons coconut aminos

1 teaspoon olive oil

Preparation

In a bowl, snow peas with mushrooms, onion, aminos, oil, salt and pepper, toss well, transfer to a pan that fits your Air Fryer, introduce in the fryer and cook at 350 °F for 15 minutes.

Divide between plates and serve as a side dish

Nutrition:

Calories 175, Fat 4g, Fiber 2g, Carbs 12g, Protein 7g

86. Gold Potatoes And Bell Pepper Mix

Preparation Time: 10 minutes

Cooking Time: 25 minutes

Servings: 4

Ingredients

4 gold potatoes, cubed

1 yellow onion, chopped

2 teaspoons olive oil

1 green bell pepper, chopped

Salt and black pepper to the taste

½ teaspoon thyme, dried

Directions:

Heat up your Air Fryer at 350 ° F, add oil, heat it up, add onion, bell pepper, salt and pepper, stir and cook for 5 minutes.

Add potatoes and thyme, stir, cover and cook at 360 °F for 20 minutes.

Divide between plates and serve as a side dish.

Nutrition:

Calories 201, Fat 4g, Fiber 4g, Carbs 12g, Protein 7g

87. Delicious Potato Mix

Preparation Time: 10 minutes

Cooking Time: 25 minutes

Servings: 6

Ingredients

6 ounces jarred roasted red bell peppers, chopped

3 garlic cloves, minced

2 tablespoons parsley, chopped

Salt and black pepper to the taste

2 tablespoons chives, chopped

4 potatoes, peeled and cut into wedges

Cooking spray

Directions:

In a pan that fits your Air Fryer, combine roasted bell peppers with garlic, parsley, salt, pepper, chives, potato wedges and the oil, toss, transfer to your Air Fryer and cook at 350 °F for 25 minutes.

Divide between plates and serve as a side dish.

Nutrition:

Calories 212, Fat 6g, Fiber 4g, Carbs 11g, Protein 5g

88. Long Beans Mix

Preparation Time: 10 minutes

Cooking Time: 10 minutes

Servings: 3

Ingredients

½ teaspoon coconut aminos

1 tablespoon olive oil

A pinch of salt and black pepper

4 garlic cloves, minced

4 long beans, trimmed and sliced

Directions:

In a pan that fits your Air Fryer, combine long beans with oil, aminos, salt, pepper and garlic, toss, introduce in your Air Fryer and cook at 350° F for 10 minutes.

Divide between plates and serve as a side dish.

Nutrition:

Calories 170, Fat 3g, Fiber 3g, Carbs 7g, Protein 3g

89. Easy Portobello Mushrooms

Preparation Time: 10 minutes

Cooking Time: 12 minutes

Servings: 4

Ingredients

4 big Portobello mushroom caps

1 tablespoon olive oil

1 cup spinach, torn

1/3 cup vegan breadcrumbs

¼ teaspoon rosemary, chopped

Preparation

Rub mushrooms caps with the oil, place them in your Air Fryer's basket and cook them at 350 ° F for 2 minutes.

Meanwhile, in a bowl, mix spinach, rosemary and breadcrumbs and stir well.

Stuff mushrooms with this mix, place them in your Air Fryer's basket again and cook at 350 ° F for 10 minutes.

Divide them between plates and serve as a side dish.

Nutrition:

Calories 152, Fat 4g, Fiber 7g, Carbs 9g, Protein 5g

90. Summer Squash Mix

Preparation Time: 10 minutes

Cooking Time: 10

Servings: 4

Ingredients

3 ounces coconut cream

½ teaspoon oregano, dried

Salt and black pepper

1 big yellow summer squash, peeled and cubed

1/3 cup carrot, cubed

2 tablespoons olive oil

Directions:

In a pan that fits your Air Fryer, combine squash with carrot, oil, oregano, salt, pepper and coconut cream, toss, transfer to your Air Fryer and cook at 400 ° F for 10 minutes.

Divide between plates and serve as a side dish.

Nutrition:

Calories 170, Fat 4g, Fiber 7g, Carbs 8g, Protein 6g

91. Leeks Medley

Preparation Time: 10 minutes

Cooking Time: 12 minutes

Servings: 4

Ingredients

6 leeks, roughly chopped

1 tablespoon cumin, ground

1 tablespoon mint, chopped

1 tablespoon parsley, chopped

1 teaspoon garlic, minced

A drizzle of olive oil

Salt and black pepper to the taste

Directions:

In a pan that fits your Air Fryer, combine leeks with cumin, mint, parsley, garlic, salt, pepper and the oil, toss, introduce in your Air Fryer and cook at 350 ° F for 12 minutes.

Divide leeks medley between plates and serve as a side dish.

Nutrition:

Calories 131, Fat 7g, Fiber 3g, Carbs 10g, Protein 6g

92. Corn And Tomatoes

Preparation Time: 10 minutes

Cooking Time: 13 minutes

Servings: 4

Ingredients

2 cups corn

4 tomatoes, roughly chopped

1 tablespoon olive oil

Salt and black pepper to the taste

1 tablespoon oregano, chopped

1 tablespoon parsley, chopped

2 tablespoons soft tofu, pressed and crumbled

Preparation

In a pan that fits your Air Fryer, combine corn with tomatoes, oil, salt, pepper, oregano and parsley, toss, introduce the pan in your Air Fryer and cook at 320 ° F for 10 minutes.

Add tofu, toss, introduce in the fryer for 3 minutes more, divide between plates and serve as a side dish.

Nutrition:

Calories 171, Fat 7g, Fiber 8g, Carbs 9g, Protein 6g

93. Broccoli, Tomatoes And Carrots

Preparation Time: 10 minutes

Cooking Time: 14 minutes

Servings: 2

Ingredients

1 broccoli head, florets separated and steamed

1 tomato, chopped

3 carrots, chopped and steamed

2 ounces soft tofu, crumbled

1 teaspoon parsley, chopped

1 teaspoon thyme, chopped

Salt and black pepper to the taste

Preparation

In a pan that fits your Air Fryer, combine broccoli with tomato, carrots, thyme, parsley, salt and pepper, toss, introduce the fryer and cook at 350 ° F for 10 minutes.

Add tofu, toss, introduce in the fryer for 4 minutes more, divide between plates and serve as a side dish.

Nutrition:

Calories 174, Fat 4g, Fiber 7g, Carbs 12g, Protein 3g

Herbed Vegetable Mélange

PREPARATION TIME: 10 MINUTES

COOKING TIME: 14 TO 18 MINUTES

SERVINGS: 4

350°F ROAST

VEGAN, GLUTEN-FREE

1 red bell pepper, sliced

1 (8-ounce) package sliced mushrooms

1 yellow summer squash, sliced

3 cloves garlic, sliced

1 tablespoon olive oil

½ teaspoon dried thyme

½ teaspoon dried basil

½ teaspoon dried tarragon

1. Place the pepper, mushrooms, squash, and garlic in a medium bowl and drizzle with the olive oil. Toss, add the thyme, basil, and tarragon, and toss again.

2. Place the vegetables in the air fryer basket. Roast for 14 to 18 minutes or until the vegetables are tender.

Air Fryer tip: When you add dried herbs to an air fryer recipe, whether you're making roasted vegetables or chicken, they must stick to the food or they will just blow around the air fryer and may burn. Always coat veggies or meat with a little oil before you add herbs, then they will stay on the food and flavor it.

Nutrition: Calories: 63; Total Fat: 4g; Saturated Fat: <1g; Cholesterol: 0mg; Sodium: 10mg; Carbohydrates: 6g; Fiber: 2g; Protein: 3g

Steamed Green Veggie Trio

PREPARATION TIME: 6 MINUTES

COOKING TIME: 9 MINUTES

SERVINGS: 4

330°F STEAM

FAST, VEGAN, GLUTEN-FREE

This combination of vegetables is delicious and classic, and can be made any time of the year. Fresh broccoli and green beans are available year-round, and peas are always stocked in the frozen section of the supermarket. Serve alongside a steak or roasted chicken for a bright side dish.

2 cups broccoli florets

1 cup green beans

1 tablespoon olive oil

1 tablespoon lemon juice

1 cup frozen baby peas

2 tablespoons honey mustard

Pinch salt

Freshly ground black pepper

1. Put the broccoli and green beans in the basket of the air fryer. Put 2 tablespoons water in the air fryer pan. Sprinkle the vegetables with the olive oil and lemon juice, and toss.

2. Steam for 6 minutes, then remove the basket from the air fryer and add the peas.

3. Steam for 3 minutes or until the vegetables are hot and tender.

4. Transfer the vegetables to a serving dish and drizzle with the honey mustard and sprinkle with salt and pepper. Toss and serve.

Ingredient tip: To prepare broccoli, cut the florets off the stem. You can freeze the stem to use in stir-fries later. To prepare green beans, cut off both ends and rinse well.

Nutrition: Calories: 99; Total Fat: 4g; Saturated Fat: <1g; Cholesterol: 0mg; Sodium: 95mg; Carbohydrates: 13g; Fiber: 4g; Protein: 4g

Garlic And Sesame Carrots

PREPARATION TIME: 5 MINUTES

COOKING TIME: 16 MINUTES

SERVINGS: 4 TO 6

380°F ROAST

1 pound baby carrots

1 tablespoon sesame oil

½ teaspoon dried dill

Pinch salt

Freshly ground black pepper

6 cloves garlic, peeled

3 tablespoons sesame seeds

1. Place the baby carrots in a medium bowl. Drizzle with sesame oil, add the dill, salt, and pepper, and toss to coat well.

2. Place the carrots in the basket of the air fryer. Roast for 8 minutes, shaking the basket once during cooking time.

3. Add the garlic to the air fryer. Roast for 8 minutes, shaking the basket once during cooking time, or until the garlic and carrots are lightly browned.

4. Transfer to a serving bowl and sprinkle with the sesame seeds before serving.

Variation tip: You can cook large carrots, cut into chunks, in place of the baby carrots in this recipe. Or you can try roasting other root vegetables, such as parsnips or rutabagas.

Nutrition: Calories: 116; Total Fat: 7g; Saturated Fat: 1g; Cholesterol: 0mg; Sodium: 129mg; Carbohydrates: 13g; Fiber: 4g; Protein: 2g

Roasted Bell Peppers With Garlic

PREPARATION TIME: 8 MINUTES

COOKING TIME: 22 MINUTES

SERVINGS: 4

330°F ROAST

1 red bell pepper

1 yellow bell pepper

1 orange bell pepper

1 green bell pepper

2 tablespoons olive oil, divided

½ teaspoon dried marjoram

Pinch salt

Freshly ground black pepper

1 head garlic

1. Slice the bell peppers into 1-inch strips.

2. In a large bowl, toss the bell peppers with 1 tablespoon of the oil. Sprinkle on the marjoram, salt, and pepper, and toss again.

3. Cut off the top of the garlic head and place the cloves on an oiled square of aluminum foil. Drizzle with the remaining olive oil. Wrap the garlic in the foil.

4. Place the wrapped garlic in the air fryer and roast for 15 minutes, then add the bell peppers. Roast for 7 minutes or until the peppers are tender and the garlic is soft. Transfer the peppers to a serving dish.

5. Remove the garlic from the air fryer and unwrap the foil. When cool enough to handle, squeeze the garlic cloves out of the papery skin and mix with the bell peppers.

Cooking tip: To easily remove the seeds from a bell pepper, cut around the stem with a sharp knife and simply pull out the stem with the seeds attached. Rinse the pepper to remove any stray seeds and cut into strips.

Nutrition: Calories: 108; Total Fat: 7g; Saturated Fat: 1g; Cholesterol: 0mg; Sodium: 45mg; Carbohydrates: 10g; Fiber: 3g; Protein: 2g

Roasted Brussels Sprouts

PREPARATION TIME: 8 MINUTES

COOKING TIME: 20 MINUTES

SERVINGS: 4

330°F ROAST

1 pound fresh Brussels sprouts

1 tablespoon olive oil

½ teaspoon salt

⅛ teaspoon pepper

¼ cup grated Parmesan cheese

1. Trim the bottoms from the Brussels sprouts and pull off any discolored leaves. Toss with the olive oil, salt, and pepper, and place in the air fryer basket.

2. Roast for 20 minutes, shaking the air fryer basket twice during cooking time, until the Brussels sprouts are dark golden brown and crisp.

3. Transfer the Brussels sprouts to a serving dish and toss with the Parmesan cheese. Serve immediately.

Did You Know? Brussels sprouts were cultivated in Roman times and introduced into the United States in the 1880s. Most Brussels sprouts in this country are grown in California.

Nutrition: Calories: 102; Total Fat: 5g; Saturated Fat: 2g; Cholesterol: 5mg; Sodium: 385mg; Carbohydrates: 11g; Fiber: 4g; Protein: 6g

Savory Roasted Sweet Potatoes

PREPARATION TIME: 5 MINUTES

COOKING TIME: 25 MINUTES

SERVINGS: 4

330°F ROAST

2 sweet potatoes, peeled and cut into 1-inch cubes

1 tablespoon olive oil

Pinch salt

Freshly ground black pepper

½ teaspoon dried thyme

½ teaspoon dried marjoram

¼ cup grated Parmesan cheese

1. Put the sweet potato cubes in the air fryer basket and drizzle with the olive oil. Toss gently. Sprinkle with the salt, pepper, thyme, and marjoram, and toss again.

2. Roast for 20 minutes, shaking the air fryer basket once during cooking time.

3. Remove the basket from the air fryer and shake the potatoes again. Sprinkle evenly with the Parmesan cheese and return to the air fryer.

4. Roast for 5 minutes or until the potatoes are tender.

Did You Know? Sweet potatoes and yams are two different types of root vegetable. A true yam is a starchy white root vegetable used in Caribbean cooking. Sweet potatoes are high in vitamin A and are usually bright orange in color.

Nutrition: Calories: 186; Total Fat: 5g; Saturated Fat: 2g; Cholesterol: 5mg; Sodium: 115mg; Carbohydrates: 32g; Fiber: 5g; Protein: 4g

Crispy Parmesan French Fries

PREPARATION TIME: 5 MINUTES

COOKING TIME: 10 MINUTES

SERVINGS: 4

390°F FRY

4 cups frozen thin French fries

2 teaspoons olive oil

⅓ cup grated Parmesan cheese

½ teaspoon dried thyme

½ teaspoon dried basil

½ teaspoon salt

1. If there is any ice on the French fries, remove it. Place the French fries in the air fryer basket and drizzle with the olive oil. Toss gently.

2. Air-fry for about 10 minutes, or until the fries are golden brown and hot, shaking the basket once during cooking time.

3. Immediately put the fries into a serving bowl and sprinkle with the Parmesan, thyme, basil, and salt. Shake to coat and serve hot.

Ingredient tip: Russet potatoes are the best for making French fries because they are low in moisture and bake up tender and crisp. You can use red potatoes or Yukon gold potatoes, but your results won't be quite as crisp.

Nutrition: Calories: 152; Total Fat: 4g; Saturated Fat: 2g; Cholesterol: 6mg; Sodium: 382mg; Carbohydrates: 24g; Fiber: 4g; Protein: 5g

Scalloped Potatoes

PREPARATION TIME: 5 MINUTES

COOKING TIME: 20 MINUTES

SERVINGS: 4

380°F BAKE

2 cups pre-sliced refrigerated potatoes

3 cloves garlic, minced

Pinch salt

Freshly ground black pepper

¾ cup heavy cream

1. Layer the potatoes, garlic, salt, and pepper in a 6-by-6-by-2-inch baking pan. Slowly pour the cream over all.

2. Bake for 15 minutes, until the potatoes are golden brown on top and tender. Check their state and, if needed, bake for 5 minutes until browned.

Ingredient tip: You can top these potatoes with cheese after about 10 minutes of baking time. Add ⅔ cup of shredded Swiss, Havarti, or Gouda, and bake until the cheese is bubbling and starts to brown.

Nutrition: Calories: 133; Total Fat: 8g; Saturated Fat: 5g; Cholesterol: 31mg; Sodium: 52mg; Carbohydrates: 13g; Fiber: 2g; Protein: 2g

Roasted Potato Salad

PREPARATION TIME: 5 MINUTES

COOKING TIME: 25 MINUTES

SERVINGS: 4 TO 6

350°F ROAST

2 pounds tiny red or creamer potatoes, cut in half

1 tablespoon plus ⅓ cup olive oil

Pinch salt

Freshly ground black pepper

1 red bell pepper, chopped

2 green onions, chopped

⅓ cup lemon juice

3 tablespoons Dijon or yellow mustard

1. Place the potatoes in the air fryer basket and drizzle with 1 tablespoon of the olive oil. Sprinkle with salt and pepper.

2. Roast for 25 minutes, shaking twice during cooking time, until the potatoes are tender and light golden brown.

3. Meanwhile, place the bell pepper and green onions in a large bowl.

4. In a small bowl, combine the remaining ⅓ cup of olive oil, the lemon juice, and mustard, and mix well with a whisk.

5. When the potatoes are cooked, add them to the bowl with the bell peppers and top with the dressing. Toss gently to coat.

6. Let cool for 20 minutes. Stir gently again and serve or refrigerate and serve later.

Variation tip: You can brighten and add complexity to this dish by adding lots of fresh chopped herbs. Try chopped dill, basil, or rosemary, depending on your preference. The warmth of the potatoes will deepen the herbs' flavor.

Nutrition: Calories: 353; Total Fat: 21g; Saturated Fat: 3g; Cholesterol: 0mg; Sodium: 192mg; Carbohydrates: 39g; Fiber: 7g; Protein: 5g

Creamy Corn Casserole

PREPARATION TIME: 5 MINUTES

COOKING TIME: 15 MINUTES

SERVINGS: 4

320°F BAKE

Nonstick baking spray with flour

2 cups frozen yellow corn

3 tablespoons flour

1 egg, beaten

¼ cup milk

½ cup light cream

½ cup grated Swiss or Havarti cheese

Pinch salt

Freshly ground black pepper

2 tablespoons butter, cut in cubes

1. Spray a 6-by-6-by-2-inch baking pan with nonstick spray.

2. In a medium bowl, combine the corn, flour, egg, milk, and light cream, and mix until combined. Stir in the cheese, salt, and pepper.

3. Pour this mixture into the prepared baking pan. Dot with the butter.

4. Bake for 15 minutes.

Substitution tip: You can substitute one 15-ounce can of corn, drained, for the frozen corn. Or cut the kernels off 2 to 3 ears of corn to use in this recipe.

Nutrition: Calories: 255; Total Fat: 16g; Saturated Fat: 10g; Cholesterol: 87mg; Sodium: 136mg; Carbohydrates: 21g; Fiber: 2g; Protein: 9g

Chapter 5 Breakfast Recipes

94. Cranberry Coconut Quinoa

Preparation Time: 10 minutes

Cooking time: 13 minutes

Servings: 4

Ingredients:

1 cup quinoa

3 cups coconut water

1 teaspoon vanilla extract

3 teaspoons stevia

1/8 cup coconut flakes

¼ cup cranberries, dried

1/8 cup almonds, chopped

Directions:

In your air fryer, mix quinoa with coconut water, vanilla, stevia, coconut flakes, almonds and cranberries, toss, cover and cook at 365 degrees F for 13 minutes.

Divide into bowls and serve for breakfast.

Enjoy!

Nutrition: calories 146, fat 5, fiber 5, carbs 10, protein 7

95. Sweet Quinoa Mix

Preparation Time: 10 minutes

Cooking time: 14 minutes

Servings: 6

Ingredients:

½ cup quinoa

1 and ½ cups steel cut oats

4 tablespoons stevia

4 and ½ cups almond milk

2 tablespoons maple syrup

1 and ½ teaspoons vanilla extract

Strawberries, halved for serving

Cooking spray

Directions:

Spray your air fryer with cooking spray, add oats, quinoa, stevia, almond milk, maple syrup and vanilla extract, toss, cover and cook at 365 degrees F for 14 minutes

Divide into bowls, add strawberries on top and serve for breakfast.

Enjoy!

Nutrition: calories 207, fat 5, fiber 8, carbs 14, protein 5

96. Chia Pudding

Preparation Time: 10 minutes

Cooking time: 15 minutes

Servings: 4

Ingredients:

1 cup chia seeds

2 cups coconut milk

2 tablespoons coconut, shredded and unsweetened

¼ cup maple syrup

½ teaspoon cinnamon powder

2 teaspoons cocoa powder

½ teaspoon vanilla extract

Directions:

In your air fryer, mix chia seeds, coconut milk, coconut, maple syrup, cinnamon, cocoa powder and vanilla, toss, cover and cook at 365 degrees F for 15 minutes

Divide chia pudding into bowls and serve for breakfast.

Enjoy!

Nutrition: calories 261, fat 4, fiber 8, carbs 10, protein 4

97. Simple Creamy Breakfast Potatoes

Preparation Time: 10 minutes

Cooking time: 20 minutes

Servings: 8

Ingredients:

Cooking spray

2 pounds gold potatoes, halved and sliced

1 yellow onion, cut into medium wedges

10 ounces canned vegan potato cream soup

8 ounces coconut milk

1 cup tofu, crumbled

½ cup veggie stock

Salt and black pepper to the taste

Directions:

Grease your air fryer's pan with cooking spray and arrange half of the potatoes on the bottom.

Layer onion wedges, half of the vegan cream soup, coconut milk, tofu, stock, salt and pepper.

Add the rest of the potatoes, onion wedges, cream, coconut milk, tofu and stock, cover and cook at 365 degrees F for 20 minutes.

Divide between plates and serve.

Enjoy!

Nutrition: calories 206, fat 14, fiber 4, carbs 10, protein 12

98. Sweet Potatoes Mix

Preparation Time: 10 minutes

Cooking time: 20 minutes

Servings: 10

Ingredients:

4 pounds sweet potatoes, thinly sliced

3 tablespoons stevia

½ cup orange juice

Salt and black pepper to the taste

½ teaspoon thyme, dried

½ teaspoon sage, dried

2 tablespoons olive oil

Directions:

Arrange potato slices on the bottom of your air fryer's pan.

In a bowl, mix orange juice with salt, pepper, stevia, thyme, sage and oil and whisk well.

Add this over potatoes, cover and cook at 365 degrees F for 20 minutes

Divide between plates and serve for breakfast

Enjoy!

Nutrition: calories 189, fat 4, fiber 4, carbs 16, protein 4

99. Breakfast Bowls

Preparation Time: 10 minutes

Cooking time: 15 minutes

Servings: 4

Ingredients:

1 block firm tofu, cut into thin strips

1 teaspoon turmeric powder

¼ cup coconut aminos

½ teaspoon onion powder

½ cup nutritional yeast

2 tablespoons olive oil

1 avocado, peeled, cored and sliced

A handful cherry tomatoes, halved

2 green onions, chopped

Salt and black pepper to the taste

Directions:

In a bowl, mix tofu strips with turmeric, coconut aminos, onion powder, half of the oil and yeast and toss.

Transfer this to your preheated air fryer at 370 degrees F and cook for 15 minutes.

In a large bowl, mix tomatoes with green onions, salt and pepper and toss.

Add tofu and the rest of the oil, toss, divide between plates and serve for breakfast.

Enjoy!

Nutrition: calories 200, fat 4, fiber 6, carbs 14, protein 5

100. Mediterranean Chickpeas Breakfast

Preparation Time: 10 minutes

Cooking time: 12 minutes

Servings: 2

Ingredients:

Cooking spray

3 shallots, chopped

2 garlic cloves, minced

½ teaspoon sweet paprika

½ teaspoon smoked paprika

½ teaspoon cinnamon powder

Salt and black pepper to the taste

2 tomatoes, chopped

2 cup chickpeas, cooked

1 tablespoon parsley, chopped

Directions:

Spray your air fryer with cooking spray and preheat it to 365 degrees F.

Add shallots, garlic, sweet and smoked paprika, cinnamon, salt, pepper, tomatoes, parsley and chickpeas, toss, cover and cook for 12 minutes.

Divide into bowls and serve for breakfast.

Enjoy!

Nutrition: calories 200, fat 4, fiber 6, carbs 12, protein 5

101. Pumpkin Breakfast Muffins

Preparation Time: 10 minutes

Cooking time: 10 minutes

Servings: 2

Ingredients:

1 and ½ cups rolled oats

½ cup pumpkin, peeled and cubed

¼ cup maple syrup

1 teaspoon cinnamon powder

¼ teaspoon nutmeg, ground

¼ teaspoon ginger powder

1/3 cup cranberries

Directions:

In your blender, mix oats with pumpkin, maple syrup, cinnamon, ginger and nutmeg and pulse well.

Fold cranberries into the mix, spoon the whole mix into muffin cups, place them in your air fryer's basket, cover and cook at 360 degrees F for 10 minutes.

Serve them for breakfast.

Enjoy!

Nutrition: calories 192, fat 4, fiber 5, carbs 14, protein 2

102. Delicious Porridge

Preparation Time: 10 minutes

Cooking time: 16 minutes

Servings: 4

Ingredients:

3 cups brown rice, cooked

1 and ¾ cups almond milk

2 tablespoons coconut sugar

2 tablespoons flaxseed meal

2 tablespoons raisins

¼ teaspoon cinnamon powder

¼ teaspoon vanilla extract

Directions:

In your air fryer, mix rice, milk, sugar, flax meal, raisins, cinnamon and vanilla, stir, cover and cook at 360 degrees F for 16 minutes.

Stir porridge again, divide into bowls and serve for breakfast.

Enjoy!

Nutrition: calories 221, fat 4, fiber 6, carbs 11, protein 4

103. Strawberry Quinoa

Preparation Time: 10 minutes

Cooking time: 10 minutes

Servings: 1

Ingredients:

¾ cup water

1 cup strawberries, halved

¼ cup cashews

1 stevia packet

1 cup quinoa

Directions:

In your air fryer's pan, mix water with cashews, quinoa and stevia, stir, cover and cook at 400 degrees F for 10 minutes.

Add strawberries, stir, divide into bowls and serve for breakfast.

Enjoy!

Nutrition: calories 177, fat 2, fiber 5, carbs 10, protein 4

104. Breakfast Broccoli And Tofu Bowls

Preparation Time: 10 minutes

Cooking time: 15 minutes

Servings: 4

Ingredients:

1 block firm tofu, pressed and cubed

1 teaspoon rice vinegar

2 tablespoons coconut aminos

1 tablespoon olive oil

1 cup quinoa, cooked

4 cups broccoli florets

2 tablespoons vegan avocado pesto

Directions:

In a bowl, mix tofu cubes with vinegar, coconut aminos, oil and broccoli, toss and leave aside for 10 minutes.

Transfer tofu to your air fryer's basket and cook at 400 degrees F for 10 minutes.

Add broccoli, cover fryer again and cook for 5 minutes more.

Divide quinoa into bowls, add tofu and broccoli, top with avocado pesto and serve for breakfast.

Enjoy!

Nutrition: calories 188, fat 3, fiber 5, carbs 8, protein 2

105. Cool Tofu Breakfast Mix

Preparation Time: 10 minutes

Cooking time: 10 minutes

Servings: 1

Ingredients:

3 ounces firm tofu, pressed and crumbled

1 cup kale, torn

½ cup broccoli florets

½ cup mushrooms, halved

¼ cup cherry tomatoes, halved

½ cup carrot, grated

¼ teaspoon garlic powder

¼ teaspoon onion powder

½ teaspoon yellow curry powder

¼ teaspoon sweet paprika

Salt and black pepper to the taste

Cooking spray

¼ cup micro greens

Directions:

Heat up your air fryer at 380 degrees F, grease its pan with cooking spray, add tofu, kale, broccoli, mushrooms, tomatoes, carrot, garlic powder, onion powder, curry powder, paprika, salt and pepper, toss, cover and cook for 10 minutes.

Divide between plates, add micro greens, toss and serve.

Enjoy!

Nutrition: calories 199, fat 2, fiber 5, carbs 12, protein 3

106. Cinnamon Oatmeal

Preparation Time: 10 minutes

Cooking time: 15 minutes

Servings: 3

Ingredients:

3 cups water

1 cup steel cut oats

1 apple, cored and chopped

1 tablespoon cinnamon powder

Directions:

In your air fryer, mix water with oats, cinnamon and apple, stir, cover and cook at 365 degrees F for 15 minutes.

Stir again, divide into bowls and serve for breakfast.

Enjoy!

Nutrition: calories 200, fat 1, fiber 7, carbs 12, protein 10

107. Coconut Rice

Preparation Time: 10 minutes

Cooking time: 15 minutes

Servings: 4

Ingredients:

1 cup Arborio rice

2 cups almond milk

1 cup coconut milk

1/3 cup agave nectar

2 teaspoons vanilla extract

¼ cup coconut flakes, toasted

Directions:

In your air fryer, mix rice with almond milk, coconut milk, agave nectar, vanilla extract and coconut flakes, cover and cook at 360 degrees F for 15 minutes.

Divide into bowls and serve warm.

Enjoy!

Nutrition: calories 192, fat 1, fiber 1, carbs 20, protein 4

108. Potato Hash

Servings: 4

Preparation Time: 15 minutes

Cooking Time: 40 minutes

Ingredients:

750 grams potatoes, washed, peeled or unpeeled, cut into small-sized cubes

250 milliliters egg substitute

3-5 tablespoons coconut oil, OR vegan fat of choice

1/2 teaspoon thyme

1/2 teaspoon savory seasoning mixture

1/2 teaspoon black pepper

1/2 green pepper, washed, seeded, and chopped

1 teaspoon salt substitute

1 onion, medium-sized, peeled and diced

Directions:

Preheat the air fryer to 180C.

Toss the green pepper and onion with half of the coconut oil and put into the air fryer basket. Set the timer for 5 minutes.

Toss the potatoes with the remaining coconut oil and the seasonings. When the air fryer timer beeps, add the potatoes in the air fryer basket, toss the ingredients to mix and cook for 30 minutes. Shake the basket after 15 minutes.

While the potato mixture is cooking in the air fryer, lightly grease a nonstick pan with cooking spray. Grind some whole peppers into the pan and let heat for 1 minutes to develop the flavor. Add the egg substitute and cook until solid. Remove from the pan, chop, and set aside.

When the air fryer timer beeps, add the egg to the air fryer basket and set the timer for 5 minutes.

Serve while piping hot with fresh tomato slices and whatever you want for breakfast.

109. French Fries

Servings: 1

Preparation Time: 5 minutes

Cooking Time: 30 minutes

Ingredients:

250 grams (9 ounces) potato

1 teaspoon coconut oil

Directions:

Wash the potatoes clean. Leave unpeeled or peel them, if preferred, and then cut into fries.

Toss the potato pieces with the coconut oil. Set the temperature to 160C or 320F and set the timer for 20-25 minutes. Halfway through cooking, shake the basket, set the temperature to 180C, and continue cooking.

110. Air-Grilled Tomatoes

Servings: 2

Preparation Time: 5 minutes

Cooking Time: 20 minutes

Ingredients:

2 tomatoes

Your preferred herbs

Ground black pepper, such as sage, rosemary, thyme, basil, oregano, parsley, etc.

Cooking spray

Directions:

Wash the tomatoes clean and then slice into halves. Spray both sides of the tomatoes with1 spray cooking spray. Sprinkle the cut portion with black pepper and your choice of fresh or dried herbs.

With the cut side faced up, put the tomato halves in the air fryer basket. Set the temperature to 160C and the timer for 20 minutes.

When the timer beeps, check the doneness, and if needed, cook for a couple of minutes. Cooking time will vary on the size and ripeness of the tomatoes and your preference.

Serve them piping hot, at room temperature, or chilled as part of an antipasto.

111. Roasted Tofu Broccoli Bowl With Quinoa

Servings: 4

Preparation Time: 30 minutes, plus 20 minutes marinating

Cooking Time: 15-17 minutes

Ingredients:

For the broccoli-tofu bowl:

1 1/4 cups water, plus more if needed for cooking the quinoa

1 block tofu, extra firm, pressed and then sliced into 1-inch cubes

1 cup quinoa

1 tablespoon olive oil

1 teaspoon rice vinegar

2 tablespoons soy sauce

4 cups broccoli florets

4 cups water

Oil-free vegan avocado pesto, ingredient and directions follow

For the oil-free vegan avocado pesto:

1 cup raw cashews

2 fresh lemons, juice only

2 Haas avocados, peels and pits removed, avocado meat chopped into pieces

2 packed cups fresh basil leaves

4 cloves garlic

Salt and pepper, to taste

Directions:

For the broccoli-tofu bowl:

Put the tofu into a large-sized, shallow dish. Add the vinegar, soy sauce, and 1 tablespoon olive oil and toss to coat. Set aside and let marinate for at least 20 minutes.

While the tofu is marinating, cook the quinoa with the 1 1/4 cups of water using the method of your choice.

Meanwhile, pour 4 cups water into a small-sized pan and bring to a boil over high heat. When the water is boiling, drop the broccoli in the water and cook for 2 minutes – don't bring back to a boil; start counting down as soon as you drop the broccoli in the hot water. After 2 minutes, immediately strain the broccoli in a colander set in the sink. Rinse immediately with cold water to stop cooking.

Transfer the marinated tofu into the air fryer basket- reserve any marinade left in the bowl. Set the temperature to 400F and the timer for 10 minutes – shake after 7 minutes.

Meanwhile, add the reserved marinade into the bowl with broccoli and toss to coat.

After the 10 minutes of tofu cooking time is over, add the broccoli to the air fryer and cook at 400F for 5 to 7 minutes.

Divide the quinoa between 4 serving bowls and divide the broccoli-tofu mixture between the bowls. Drizzle the top with the pesto or your preferred sauce.

For the oil-free vegan avocado pesto:

Put all of the ingredients in a blender and blend until smooth – add 1 tablespoon water at a time as needed to get the ingredients moving. Season with pepper and salt to taste.

You can use this as a sandwich spread, over pasta, or with veggies or bread.

Notes: You can make the pesto while the broccoli and tofu cook. Use any sauce if you do not like pesto.

112. Breakfast-Style Potatoes

Servings: 2-4

Preparation Time: 10 minutes

Cooking Time: 25 minutes

Ingredients:

2 Russet potatoes, medium- sized, (about 13 ounces or 2 generous cups total), chopped into roughly 1-inch pieces

1 onion, small-sized (about 4 ounces or 3/4 cup), chopped into medium-sized pieces

1 bell pepper, small-sized, (about 5 ounces or 3/4 cup), chopped into medium-sized pieces

A couple generous sprays of cooking oil spray

Pinch salt and pepper

Directions:

Put the potatoes in the air fryer basket. Spray with cooking oil spray, shake, spray again, and sprinkle with 1 pinch salt.

Set the temperature to 400F and set the timer for 10 minutes. Stop halfway during cooking to shake or stir the potatoes and continue during cooking.

When the ten minutes are up, add the onions and bell pepper in the air fryer. Spray with cooking oil and shake the basket. Cook at 400F for another 15 minutes. When there are only 5 minutes left in the cooking time, check the potatoes to ensure that they are not browning too much – cooking time will depend on the size of the potatoes. Add a couple more cooking time, if needed. Season with salt to taste and then serve.

113. Hot Polenta Rounds

Servings: 4

Preparation Time: 10 minutes

Cooking Time: 35 minutes

Ingredients:

1 package (18 ounces) pre-cooked ancient-harvest polenta roll

1 tablespoon extra-virgin olive oil

Directions:

Open the package of polenta roll. Using a sharp knife, slice the polenta into 1/2-inch thick round slices. Brush all the sides of the polenta slices with the olive oil.

Apply cooking oil onto the air fryer basket and preheat at 400F for 5 minutes.

Put the polenta slices in the basket and set the timer for 25 minutes. When the timer beeps, flip the slices and cook for 5-10 minutes more.

Chapter 6 Lunch Recipes

114. Corn And Cabbage Salad

Preparation Time: 10 minutes

Cooking time: 15 minutes

Servings: 4

Ingredients:

1 small yellow onion, chopped

1 tablespoon olive oil

2 garlic cloves, minced

1 and ½ cups mushrooms, sliced

3 teaspoons ginger, grated

A pinch of salt and black pepper

2 cups corn

4 cups red cabbage, chopped

1 tablespoon nutritional yeast

2 teaspoons tomato paste

1 teaspoon coconut aminos

1 teaspoon sriracha sauce

Directions:

In your air fryer's pan, mix the oil with onion, garlic, mushrooms, ginger, salt, pepper, corn, cabbage, yeast and tomato paste, stir, cover and cook at 365 degrees F for 15 minutes

Add sriracha sauce and aminos, stir, divide between plates and serve.

Enjoy!

Nutrition: calories 360, fat 4, fiber 4, carbs 10, protein 4

115. Okra And Corn Mix

Preparation Time: 10 minutes

Cooking time: 15 minutes

Servings: 6

Ingredients:

1 green bell pepper, chopped

1 small yellow onion, chopped

3 garlic cloves, minced

16 ounces okra, sliced

2 cup corn

12 ounces canned tomatoes, crushed

1 and ½ teaspoon smoked paprika

1 teaspoon marjoram, dried

1 teaspoon thyme, dried

1 teaspoon oregano, dried

Salt and black pepper to the taste

Directions:

In your air fryer, mix bell pepper with onion, garlic, okra, corn, tomatoes, smoked paprika, marjoram, thyme, oregano, salt and pepper, stir, cover and cook at 360 degrees F for 15 minutes.

Stir, divide between plates and serve.

Enjoy!

Nutrition: calories 243, fat 4, fiber 6, carbs 10, protein 3

116. Potato And Carrot Mix

Preparation Time: 10 minutes

Cooking time: 16 minutes

Servings: 6

Ingredients:

2 potatoes, cubed

3 pounds carrots, cubed

1 yellow onion, chopped

Salt and black pepper to the taste

1 teaspoon thyme, dried

3 tablespoons coconut milk

2 teaspoons curry powder

3 tablespoons vegan cheese, crumbled

1 tablespoon parsley, chopped

Directions:

In your air fryer's pan, mix onion with potatoes, carrots, salt, pepper, thyme and curry powder, stir, cover and cook at 365 degrees F for 16 minutes.

Add coconut milk, sprinkle vegan cheese, divide between plates and serve.

Enjoy!

Nutrition: calories 241, fat 4, fiber 7, carbs 8, protein 4

117. Winter Green Beans

Preparation Time: 10 minutes

Cooking time: 16 minutes

Servings: 4

Ingredients:

1 and ½ cups yellow onion, chopped

1 pound green beans, halved

4 ounces canned tomatoes, chopped

4 garlic cloves, chopped

2 teaspoons oregano, dried

1 jalapeno, chopped

Salt and black pepper to the taste

1 and ½ teaspoons cumin, ground

1 tablespoons olive oil

Directions:

Preheat your air fryer to 365 degrees F, add oil to the pan, also add onion, green beans, tomatoes, garlic, oregano, jalapeno, salt, pepper and cumin, cover and cook for 16 minutes.

Divide between plates and serve.

Enjoy!

Nutrition: calories 261, fat 5, fiber 8, carbs 10, protein 12

118. Green Beans Casserole

Preparation Time: 10 minutes

Cooking time: 20 minutes

Servings: 4

Ingredients:

1 teaspoon olive oil

2 red chilies, dried

¼ teaspoon fenugreek seeds

½ teaspoon black mustard seeds

10 curry leaves, chopped

½ cup red onion, chopped

3 garlic cloves, minced

2 teaspoons coriander powder

2 tomatoes, chopped

2 cups eggplant, chopped

½ teaspoon turmeric powder

½ cup green bell pepper, chopped

A pinch of salt and black pepper

1 cup green beans, trimmed and halved

2 teaspoons tamarind paste

1 tablespoons cilantro, chopped

Directions:

In a baking dish that fits your air fryer, combine oil with chilies, fenugreek seeds, black mustard seeds, curry leaves, onion, coriander, tomatoes, eggplant, turmeric, green bell pepper, salt, pepper, green beans, tamarind paste and cilantro, toss, put in your air fryer and cook at 365 degrees F for 20 minutes.

Divide between plates and serve.

Nutrition: calories 251, fat 5, fiber 4, carbs 8, protein 12

119. Chipotle Green Beans

Preparation Time: 10 minutes

Cooking time: 16 minutes

Servings: 6

Ingredients:

1 yellow onion, chopped

1 pound green beans, halved

2 teaspoons cumin, ground

A drizzle of olive oil

12 ounces corn

¼ teaspoon chipotle powder

1 cup salsa

Directions:

In a pan that fits your air fryer, combine oil with onion, green beans, cumin, corn, chipotle powder and salsa, toss, introduce in your air fryer and cook at 365 degrees F for 16 minutes.

Divide between plates and serve.

Enjoy!

Nutrition: calories 224, fat 2, fiber 12, carbs 14, protein 10

120. Cranberry Beans Pasta

Preparation Time: 10 minutes

Cooking time: 15 minutes

Servings: 8

Ingredients:

2 cups canned cranberry beans, drained

2 celery ribs, chopped

1 yellow onion, chopped

7 garlic cloves, minced

1 teaspoon rosemary, chopped

26 ounces canned tomatoes, chopped

¼ teaspoon red pepper flakes

2 teaspoons oregano, dried

3 teaspoons basil, dried

½ teaspoon smoked paprika

A pinch of salt and black pepper

10 ounces kale, roughly chopped

2 cups whole wheat vegan pasta, cooked

Directions:

In a pan that fits your air fryer, combine beans with celery, onion, garlic, rosemary, tomatoes, pepper flakes, oregano, basil, paprika, salt, pepper and kale, introduce in your air fryer and cook at 365 degrees F for 15 minutes.

Divide vegan pasta between plates, add cranberry mix on top and serve.

Enjoy!

Nutrition: calories 251, fat 2, fiber 12, carbs 12, protein 6

121. Mexican Casserole

Preparation Time: 10 minutes

Cooking time: 15 minutes

Servings: 4

Ingredients:

1 tablespoon olive oil

4 garlic cloves, minced

1 yellow onion, chopped

2 tablespoons cilantro, chopped

1 small red chili, chopped

2 teaspoons cumin, ground

Salt and black pepper to the taste

1 teaspoon sweet paprika

1 teaspoon coriander seeds

1 pound sweet potatoes, cubed

Juice of ½ lime

10 ounces green beans

2 cups tomatoes, chopped

1 tablespoon parsley, chopped

Directions:

Grease a pan that fits your air fryer with the oil, add garlic, onion, cilantro, red chili, cumin, salt, pepper, paprika, coriander, potatoes, lime juice, green beans and tomatoes, toss, place in your air fryer and cook at 365 degrees F for 15 minutes.

Add parsley, divide between plates and serve.

Enjoy!

Nutrition: calories 223, fat 5, fiber 4, carbs 7, protein 8

122. Endives And Rice Casserole

Preparation Time: 10 minutes

Cooking time: 20 minutes

Servings: 4

Ingredients:

1 tablespoon olive oil

2 scallions, chopped

3 garlic cloves chopped

1 tablespoon ginger, grated

1 teaspoon chili sauce

A pinch of salt and black pepper

½ cup white rice

1 cup veggie stock

3 endives, trimmed and chopped

Directions:

Grease a pan that fits your air fryer with the oil, add scallions, garlic, ginger, chili sauce, salt, pepper, rice, stock and endives, place in your air fryer, cover and cook at 365 degrees F for 20 minutes.

Divide casserole between plates and serve.

Enjoy!

Nutrition: calories 220, fat 5, fiber 8, carbs 12, protein 6

123. Cabbage And Tomatoes

Preparation Time: 10 minutes

Cooking time: 12 minutes

Servings: 4

Ingredients:

1 tablespoon olive oil

1 green cabbage head, chopped

Salt and black pepper to the taste

15 ounces canned tomatoes, chopped

½ cup yellow onion, chopped

2 teaspoons turmeric powder

Directions:

In a pan that fits your air fryer, combine oil with green cabbage, salt, pepper, tomatoes, onion and turmeric, place in your air fryer and cook at 365 degrees F for 12 minutes.

Divide between plates and serve.

Enjoy!

Nutrition: calories 202, fat 5, fiber 8, carbs 9, protein 10

124. Simple Endive Mix

Preparation Time: 10 minutes

Cooking time: 10 minutes

Servings: 4

Ingredients:

8 endives, trimmed

Salt and black pepper to the taste

3 tablespoons olive oil

Juice of ½ lemon

1 tablespoon tomato paste

2 tablespoons parsley, chopped

1 teaspoon stevia

Directions:

In a bowl, combine endives with salt, pepper, oil, lemon juice, tomato paste, parsley and stevia, toss, place endives in your air fryer's basket and cook at 365 degrees F for 10 minutes.

Divide between plates and serve.

Enjoy!

Nutrition: calories 160, fat 4, fiber 7, carbs 9, protein 4

125. Eggplant And Tomato Sauce

Preparation Time: 10 minutes

Cooking time: 12 minutes

Servings: 2

Ingredients:

4 cups eggplant, cubed

1 tablespoon olive oil

1 tablespoon garlic powder

A pinch of salt and black pepper

3 garlic cloves, minced

1 cup tomato sauce

Directions:

In a pan that fits your air fryer, combine eggplant cubes with oil, garlic, salt, pepper, garlic powder and tomato sauce, toss, place in your air fryer and cook at 370 degrees F for 12 minutes.

Divide between plates and serve.

Enjoy!

Nutrition: calories 250, fat 7, fiber 5, carbs 10, protein 4

126. Brown Rice And Mung Beans Mix

Preparation Time: 10 minutes

Cooking time: 16 minutes

Servings: 2

Ingredients:

½ teaspoon olive oil

½ cup brown rice, cooked

½ cup mung beans

½ teaspoon cumin seeds

½ cup red onion, chopped

2 tomatoes, chopped

1 small ginger piece, grated

4 garlic cloves, minced

1 teaspoon coriander, ground

½ teaspoon turmeric powder

A pinch of cayenne pepper

½ teaspoon garam masala

1 cup veggie stock

Salt and black pepper to the taste

1 teaspoon lemon juice

Directions:

In your blender, mix tomato with garlic, onions, ginger, salt, pepper, garam masala, cayenne, coriander and turmeric and pulse really well.

In a pan that fits your air fryer, combine oil with blended tomato mix, mung beans, rice, stock, cumin and lemon juice, place in your air fryer and cook at 365 degrees F for 16 minutes.

Divide everything between plates and serve.

Enjoy!

Nutrition: calories 200, fat 6, fiber 7, carbs 10, protein 8

127. Lentils And Spinach Casserole

Preparation Time: 10 minutes

Cooking time: 16 minutes

Servings: 3

Ingredients:

1 teaspoon olive oil

1/3 cup canned brown lentils, drained

1 small ginger piece, grated

4 garlic cloves, minced

1 green chili pepper, chopped

2 tomatoes, chopped

½ teaspoon garam masala

½ teaspoon turmeric powder

2 potatoes, cubed

Salt and black pepper to the taste

¼ teaspoon cardamom, ground

¼ teaspoon cinnamon powder

6 ounces spinach leaves

Directions:

In a pan that fits your air fryer combine oil with canned lentils, ginger, garlic, chili pepper, tomatoes, garam masala, turmeric, potatoes, salt, pepper, cardamom, cinnamon and spinach, toss, place in your air fryer and cook at 356 degrees F for 16 minutes.

Divide casserole between plates and serve.

Enjoy!

Nutrition: calories 250, fat 3, fiber 11, carbs 16, protein 10

128. Red Potatoes And Tasty Chutney

Preparation Time: 10 minutes

Cooking time: 14 minutes

Servings: 4

Ingredients:

2 pounds red potatoes, cubed

1 cup green beans

1 cup carrots, shredded

16 ounces canned chickpeas, drained

2 tablespoons olive oil

1 teaspoon coriander seeds

1 and ½ teaspoons cumin seeds

1 and ½ teaspoons garam masala

½ teaspoon mustard seeds

1 teaspoon garlic, minced

For the chutney:

¼ cup water

½ cup mint

½ cup cilantro

1 small ginger piece, grated

2 teaspoons lime juice

A pinch of salt

Directions:

In a baking dish that fits your air fryer, combine oil with potatoes, green beans, carrots, chickpeas, coriander, cumin, garam masala, mustard seeds and garlic, place in your air fryer and cook at 365 degrees F for 20 minutes.

In your blender, mix water with mint, cilantro, ginger, lime juice and salt and pulse really well.

Divide potato mix between plates, add mint chutney on top and serve.

Enjoy!

Nutrition: calories 241, fat 4, fiber 7, carbs 11, protein 6

129. Simple Veggie Salad

Preparation Time: 10 minutes

Cooking time: 10 minutes

Servings: 8

Ingredients:

1 and ½ cups tomatoes, chopped

3 cups eggplant, chopped

2 teaspoons capers

Cooking spray

3 garlic cloves, minced

2 teaspoons balsamic vinegar

1 tablespoon basil, chopped

A pinch of salt and black pepper

Directions:

Grease a pan that fits your air fryer with cooking spray, add tomatoes, eggplant, capers, garlic, salt and pepper, place in your air fryer and cook at 365 degrees F for 10 minutes.

Divide between plates, drizzle balsamic vinegar all over, sprinkle basil and serve cold.

Enjoy!

Nutrition: calories 171, fat 3, fiber 1, carbs 8, protein 12

130. Black Beans Veggie Burgers

Preparation Time: 20 minutes

Servings: 7

Ingredients:

One can of drained and rinsed black beans

½ a green bell pepper

½ small and cut onion

Two cloves of peeled garlic

One large egg

1 tbsp. of chili powder

1 tbsp. of cumin

1 tbsp. of Thai chili sauce or you can use hot sauce too

½ cup of bread crumbs

Directions:

Preheat your air fryer to a high heat.

In a large bowl, mash your black beans using a fork until it becomes thick and pasty.

With the utilization of a food processor, chop the pepper, the onion, and the garlic.

Stir in the mashed beans.

Now, take a small bowl and place in it, the chili powder, the cumin, and the chili sauce.

Stir in the egg mixture to the mixture of the mashed beans.

Combine the bread crumbs and keep stirring until the mixture becomes sticky.

Now, divide your mixture into some four patties.

Arrange the patties in the basket of the air fryer.

Slide the basket of the air fryer and bake it for 8 minutes on each of its sides.

Once cooked, enjoy your meal.

Nutrition

Fat: 3g

Calories: 30

Dietary Fiber: 4.6g

Protein: 7g

131. Veggie Muffins With Cheese

Preparation Time: 30 minutes

Servings: 5

Ingredients:

Five split and toasted English muffins

One mashed avocado

1 cup of alfalfa sprouts

1 chopped tomato

1 chopped sweet onion

4 tbsp. of Ranch-style salad dressing

4 tbsp. of toasted sesame seeds

1 cup of shredded and smoked Cheddar cheese

Directions:

Preheat your air fryer.

In the basket of the air fryer, arrange the muffins open faced.

Spread mashed avocado on each half of muffin.

Place the halves close to each other.

Distribute the ingredients that you have evenly on the halves of the muffins.

Cover the biscuits with sprouts, the tomatoes, the onion, the dressing, the sesame seeds and the cheese.

Set your timer for 5 minutes and the heat to 390° F and slide the basket in the air fryer.

Lock the lid and wait until the cheese melts over the muffins.

Serve and enjoy your cupcakes!

Nutrition

Fat: 3g

Calories: 34

Dietary Fiber: 3g

Protein: 2g

132. Tomato Gillette

Preparation Time: 30 minutes

Servings: 5

Ingredients:

3 Large tomatoes

A pinch of salt

A pinch of black pepper

Herbs

1tbsp of olive oil

1 cup of mozzarella cheese

Sheet of puff pastry

Directions:

Wash your tomatoes very well.

Cut the tomatoes into halves in any direction of your choice.

Heat olive oil and add the tomatoes.

Sprinkle the tomatoes with black ground black pepper.

Add dried herbs of your choice.

Add cheese above the tomatoes.

You can also use fresh herbs.

Add parsley, basil, oregano, thyme, rosemary and sage.

Set aside.

Roll out the dough to make a circle, sprinkle the cooked tomato mixture at the Centre of the dough and spread it to form a layer on the dough.

Fold the dough to form pleats, repeat the procedure.

Establish the heat to 320° F then fry.

After the timer gets off, remove your tomato Gillette's and serve them warm.

Enjoy!

Nutrition

Fat: 5g

Calories: 45

Dietary Fiber: 2g

Protein: 13g

133. Persian Mushrooms:

Preparation Time: 25 minutes

Servings: 4

Ingredients:

6 Portobello large mushrooms

3 oz of softened butter

Two large shallots

Two cloves of garlic

Fresh parsley

A pinch of salt

A pinch of pepper

1 cup of grated parmesan

Directions:

Preheat your air fryer to 390° F.

Clean your mushrooms and brush them lightly to remove any soil.

Eliminate the stems and cut the wedges of at the end of the mushrooms.

Slice your shallots and the garlic too.

Now; place your mushroom stems, the garlic and the shallots with the parsley and the softened butter in a blender.

Arrange the caps of your mushrooms in the basket of the air fryer.

Stuff the caps with your mixture and sprinkle the Parmesan cheese.

Slide the basket in the air fryer.

Set your timer to 20 minutes.

When the time goes off, serve your mushrooms hot with burgers.

Enjoy your delicious mushroom meal!

Nutrition

Fat: 4g

Calories: 45

Dietary Fiber: 2.4g

Protein: 13g

134. Stuffed Peppers With Tomato Sauce

Preparation Time: 25 minutes

Servings: 3

Ingredients:

1 cup of water (If you want to add flavor, use chicken broth)

1 cup of uncooked Arborio rice

Five large green peppers, (Make sure to halve and seed the bell peppers, or you can choose another way by cutting the stems and emptying the inner of the pepper)

1tbsp of olive oil

Three thinly sliced medium green onions

1teaspoon of dried basil

1teaspoon of Italian seasoning

One teaspoon of salt

One pinch of ground black pepper

1 Large tomato cut into cubes

½ cup of crumbled feta cheese

Directions:

Preheat your air fryer to 390° F.

Meanwhile, in a saucepan, boil the water.

Add the rice.

Lower the heat.

Place all your peppers in the basket of the air fryer.

Roast the peppers from 24 to 30 minutes in your preheated Air fryer.

Remove the peppers when it starts to get brown.

While your peppers are still being roasted, heat the oil in a skillet at a high heat.

Now reduce the heat and cook your onions.

Add the basil, the Italian seasoning, the salt, and the pepper.

Sauté the ingredients in the oil for 2 to 3 minutes.

Add the tomato; then cook for five more minutes.

Test the rice with a spoon to see if it is perfectly cooked.

Add the feta cheese.

Spoon the entire mixture into the halves of the pepper.

Return the peppers to the air fryer for 5 minutes.

Serve your peppers immediately with the tomato sauce.

Nutrition

Fat: 3g

Calories: 35

Dietary Fiber: 2g

Protein: 12g

135. Spicy Crispy Cabbage

Preparation: 30 minutes

Serving: 5

Ingredients:

A half a head of white cabbage, chopped into small pieces and washed

One tablespoon of coconut oil, melted to liquid

A pinch of sea salt

A pinch of chili, cayenne pepper, garlic powder

Directions:

In a large mixing bowl, combine the chopped cabbage with the coconut oil and the spices.

Take care that the cabbage is lightly coated.

Place the cabbage in the Air fryer basket. Fry for 10 minutes.

Serve and Enjoy!

Nutrition

Fat: 2g

Calories: 21

Dietary Fiber: 4g

Protein: 20g

136. Carrots Rice

Preparation Time: 20 minutes

Servings: 3

Ingredients:

1 Cup of basmati rice

2 Cups of water

¼ Cup of roasted peanuts

1 tbsp. of margarine

1 Sliced onion

1 Teaspoon of minced and fresh ginger root

¾ Cup of grated carrots

A pinch of salt

A pinch of black pepper

2 tbsp. of chopped cilantro

Directions:

Combine the rice and the water in a saucepan.

Boil the rice over high heat.

After 2 minutes of boiling, lower the heat.

Cover the saucepan with its lid and let it boil for around 15 to 20 minutes.

While your rice is being cooked, grind your peanuts in a processor and set it aside.

Heat the butter in the air fryer over a medium heat.

Stir in the rice, top it with the ginger, carrots then set your timer to 5 minutes.

Remove the rice from the air fryer and place it on a serving plate.

Season the rice with the salt and the black pepper; you can add peanuts if you want.

Garnish the rice with cilantro.

Serve and enjoy your delicious dish.

Nutrition

Fat: 3g

Calories: 23

Dietary Fiber: 2g

Protein: 12g

137. Air Fried Zucchini Chips

Servings: 3

Preparation Time: 20 Minutes

Calories: 187

Fat: 6.6 g

Protein: 10.8 g

Carbs: 21.1 g

Ingredients

1 cup panko bread crumbs

3/4 grated Parmesan cheese

1 medium zucchini, sliced thinly

1 large egg, beaten

Direction

Place the Ninja Foodi Cook and Crisp basket in the ceramic pot.

Mix the panko bread crumbs and parmesan cheese. Set aside.

Dip the zucchini in egg before dredging in the panko mixture.

Place the dredged zucchini in the basket.

Close the crisping lid and press the Air Crisp button before pressing the START button.

Adjust the cooking time to 15 minutes. Serve and enjoy!

138. Crispy Cauliflower Bites

Servings: 4

Preparation Time: 12 Minutes

Calories: 130

Fat: 7 g

Protein: 4.3 g

Carbs: 12.4 g

Ingredients

3 garlic cloves, minced

1 tbsp. olive oil

1/2 tsp. salt

1/2 tsp. smoked paprika

4 cups cauliflower florets

Direction

Place in the ceramic pot the Foodi Cook and Crisp basket.

Place all ingredients in a bowl and toss to combine.

Place the seasoned cauliflower florets in the basket.

Close the crisping lid and press the Air Crisp button before pressing the START button.

Adjust the cooking time to 10 minutes.

Give the basket a shake while cooking for even cooking. Serve and enjoy!

139. Baked Bananas

Servings: 4

Preparation Time: 12 Minutes

Calories: 183

Fat: 0.9 g

Protein: 1.4 g

Carbs: 42.2 g

Ingredients

4 firm bananas, peeled and halved

1/4 cup maple syrup

1 tbsp. ground cinnamon

1 piece fresh ginger, grated

1 1/2 tsp. nutmeg

Direction

Place in the ceramic pot the Foodi Cook and Crisp reversible rack.

In a bowl, season the bananas with maple syrup, ground cinnamon, ginger, and nutmeg.

Place the bananas on the rack.

Close the crisping lid and press the Bake/Roast button before pressing the START button.

Adjust the cooking time to 10 minutes. Serve and enjoy!

140. Spicy Roasted Broccoli

Servings: 2

Preparation Time: 23 Minutes

Calories: 76

Fat: 3.9 g

Protein: 2.1 g

Carbs: 8 g

Ingredients

2 cups broccoli florets

1 yellow bell pepper, sliced

1 tsp. garlic powder

1 tbsp. steak seasoning

2 tsp. chili powder

1 tbsp. extra virgin olive oil

Salt and pepper, to taste

Direction

Place in the ceramic pot the Foodi Cook and Crisp basket insert.

Toss all ingredients in a mixing bowl.

Place the vegetables in the basket.

Close the crisping lid and press the Bake/Roast button before pressing the START button.

Adjust the cooking time to 20 minutes.

Give the basket a shake to roast the veggies evenly. Serve and enjoy!

141. Quinoa And Potato Salad

Servings: 6

Preparation Time: 25 Minutes

Ingredients

1/4 cup white balsamic vinegar

1 tbsp. Dijon mustard

1 tsp. sweet paprika

1/2 tsp. ground black pepper

1/4 tsp. celery seeds

1/4 tsp. salt

1/4 cup olive oil

1 1/2 pounds tiny white potatoes, halved

1 cup blond (white) quinoa

1 medium shallot, minced

2 medium celery stalks, thinly sliced

1 large dill pickle, diced

Direction

Whisk the vinegar, mustard, paprika, pepper, celery seeds and salt in a large serving bowl until smooth.

Whisk in the olive oil in a thin, steady stream until the dressing is fairly creamy.

Place the potatoes and quinoa in the Ninja Foodi Multicooker; add enough cold tap water so that the ingredients are submerged by 3 inches (some of the quinoa may float).

Lock the lid on the Ninja Foodi Multicooker and then cook for 10 minutes. To get 10-minutes cook time, press "Pressure" button and use the Time Adjustment button to adjust the cook time to 10 minutes.

Use the quick-release method to bring the pot's pressure back to normal.

Unlock and open the pot. Close the crisping lid.

Select BROIL, and set the time to 5 minutes. Select START/STOP to begin.

Cook until top has browned.

Drain the contents of the pot into a colander lined with paper towels or into a fine-mesh sieve in the sink. Do not rinse.

Transfer the potatoes and quinoa to the large bowl with the dressing.

Add the shallot, celery, and pickle; toss gently and set aside for a minute or two to warm up the vegetables. Serve and enjoy!

142. Buttery Carrots With Pancetta

Servings: 5

Preparation Time: 20 Minutes

Ingredients

4 oz. pancetta, diced

1 medium leek, white and pale green parts only, sliced lengthwise, washed and thinly sliced

1/4 cup moderately sweet white wine (I used dry Riesling)

1 pound baby carrots

1/2 tsp. ground black pepper

2 tbsp. unsalted butter, cut into small bits

Direction

Put the pancetta in the Ninja Foodi turned to the Air Crisp function.

Use time adjustment button to set cooking time to 5 minutes.

Add the leeks; cook, often stirring, until softened.

Pour in the wine and scrape up any browned bits at the bottom of the pot as it comes to a simmer.

Add the carrots and pepper; stir well.

Scrape and pour the contents of the Ninja Foodi Multicooker into a 1-quart, round, high-sided soufflé or baking dish. Dot with the bits of butter.

Lay a piece of parchment paper on top of the dish, then a piece of aluminum foil.

Seal the foil tightly over the baking dish.

Set the Ninja Foodi Multicooker rack inside, and pour in 2 cups water.

Use aluminum foil to build a sling for the baking dish; lower the baking dish into the cooker.

Lock the lid on the Ninja Foodi Multicooker and then cook for 7 minutes. To get 7-minutes cook time, press "Pressure" button and use the Time Adjustment button to adjust the cook time to 7 minutes.

Use the quick-release method to return the pot's pressure to normal.

Close the crisping lid. Select BROIL, and set the time to 5 minutes.

Select START/STOP to begin. Cook until top has browned.

Unlock and open the pot. Use the foil sling to lift the baking dish out of the cooker.

Uncover and stir well. Serve and enjoy!

143. Braised Red Cabbage With Apples

Servings: 4

Preparation Time: 20 Minutes

Ingredients

4 thin bacon slices, chopped

1 small red onion, chopped

1 medium tart green apple (I used Granny Smith), peeled, cored and chopped

1 tsp. dried thyme

1/4 tsp. dried thyme

1/4 tsp. ground allspice

1/4 tsp. ground mace

1 tbsp. packed dark brown sugar

1 tbsp. balsamic vinegar

1 medium red cabbage (about 2 pounds), cored and thinly sliced

1/2 cup chicken broth

Direction

Fry the bacon in the Ninja Foodi turned to the Air Crisp function until crisp which takes about 4 minutes.

Add the onion to the pot; cook, often stirring, until soft, about 4 minutes.

Add the apple, thyme, allspice, and mace. Cook about 1 minute, stirring all the while, until fragrant.

Stir in the brown sugar and vinegar; keep stirring until bubbling, about 1 minute.

Add the cabbage; toss well to mix evenly with the other ingredients. Drizzle the broth over the cabbage mixture.

Lock the lid on the Ninja Foodi Multicooker and then cook for 13 minutes. To get 13-minutes cook time, press "Pressure" button, and use the Time Adjustment button to adjust the cook time to 13 minutes.

Use the quick-release method to return the pot to normal pressure.

Unlock and open the pot. Close the crisping lid.

Select BROIL, and set the time to 5 minutes.

Press the Start/Stop button to begin.

Cook until top has browned. Serve and enjoy!

144. Sage-Butter Spaghetti Squash

Servings: 6

Preparation Time: 25 Minutes

Ingredients

One 3 1/2 pound spaghetti squash

6 tbsp. unsalted butter

2 tbsp. packed fresh sage leaves, minced

1/2 tsp. salt

1/2 tsp. ground black pepper

1/2 cup finely grated Parmesan cheese (about 1 oz.)

Direction

Put the squash with the cut side facing up in the cooker. Then add 1 cup water.

Lock the lid on the Ninja Foodi and then cook for 12 minutes.

Use the quick-release method to bring the pot's pressure back to normal.

Unlock and open the cooker. Transfer the squash halves to a cutting board; cool for 10 minutes.

Discard the liquid in the cooker.

Use a fork to scrape the spaghetti-like flesh off the skin and onto the cutting board; discard the skins.

Melt the butter in the electric cooker turned to its browning function.

Stir in the sage, salt, and pepper, then add all of the squash.

Stir and toss over the heat until well combined and heated through about 2 minutes.

Add the cheese, toss well. Close the crisping lid.

Select BROIL, and set the time to 5 minutes.

Select START/STOP to begin.

Cook until top has browned. Serve and enjoy!

145. Rye Berry And Celery Root Salad

Servings: 6

Preparation Time: 45 Minutes

Ingredients

3/4 cup rye berries

1 medium celeriac (celery root), peeled and shredded through the large holes of a box grater

2 tbsp. unsalted butter

2 tbsp. honey

2 tbsp. apple cider vinegar

1/2 tsp. salt

1/2 tsp. ground black pepper

Direction

Place the rye berries in the Foodi; pour in enough cold tap water, so the grains are submerged by 2 inches.

Lock the lid on the Foodi and then cook for 40 minutes.

Pressure Release. Use the quick-release method to bring the pot's pressure back to normal.

Unlock and open the cooker. Stir in the shredded celeriac.

Cover the pot without locking it and set aside for 1 minute.

Drain the pot into a large colander set in the sink.

Wipe out the cooker. Melt the butter in the Foodi; turned to it sauté function.

Add the honey and cook for 1 minute, constantly stirring.

Add the drained rye berries and celeriac; cook, constantly stirring, for 1 minute.

Stir in the vinegar, salt, and pepper to serve. Enjoy!

146. Fried Soy Curls

Servings: 2

Preparation Time: 40 Minutes

Calories: 100

Fat: 1 g

Protein: 4 g

Carbs: 17 g

Ingredients

4 oz. soy curls

3 cups hot water

1/4 fine ground cornmeal

1/4 cup nutritional yeast

1 tsp. poultry seasoning

1 tsp. Cajun seasoning

Salt and pepper, to taste

Direction

Soak the soy curls in hot water for 10 minutes.

Drain in a strainer.

Press the water out.

In a bowl, mix the rest of the ingredients.

Coat each soy curl with the breading.

Place in the Ninja Foodi basket.

Seal the crisping lid.

Set it to air crisp function.

Cook at 380 degrees for 5 minutes.

Season with the salt and pepper.

You can serve with mashed potatoes and gravy. Enjoy!

147. Crispy Tofu

Servings: 4

Preparation Time: 60 Minutes

Calories: 137

Fat: 3.4 g

Protein: 2.3 g

Carbs: 24 g

Ingredients

1 tsp. seasoned rice vinegar

2 tbsp. low sodium soy sauce

2 tsp. toasted sesame oil

1 block firm tofu, sliced into cubes

1 tbsp. potato starch

Cooking spray

Direction

In a bowl, mix the vinegar, soy sauce, and sesame oil.

Marinate the tofu for 30 minutes.

Coat the tofu with potato starch.

Spray the Ninja Foodi basket with oil.

Seal the crisping lid.

Choose the air crisp setting.

Cook at 370 degrees for 20 minutes, flipping halfway through.

You can serve with soy sauce and vinegar dipping sauce. Enjoy!

148. Onion Rings

Servings: 4

Preparation Time: 40 Minutes

Calories: 147

Fat: 11.3 g

Protein: 2.6 g

Carbs: 10.9 g

Ingredients

3 yellow onions, sliced into rings

1/2 cup almond flour

2/3 cup unsweetened coconut milk

1/2 tsp. paprika

1/4 tsp. turmeric

Salt, to taste

Direction

Mix all the ingredients except the onion rings in a large bowl.

Coat each onion ring with the mixture.

Place in the Ninja Foodi basket.

Seal the crisping lid.

Set it to air crisp.

Cook at 400 degrees for 10 minutes, flipping halfway through.

You can serve with ketchup or hot sauce. Enjoy!

149. Potato Wedges

Servings: 4

Preparation Time: 40 Minutes

Calories: 179

Fat: 2.6 g

Protein: 2.8 g

Carbs: 36.2 g

Ingredients

1 lb. potatoes, sliced into wedges

1 tsp. olive oil

Salt and pepper, to taste

1/2 tsp. garlic powder

Direction

Coat the potatoes with oil.

Season with salt, pepper and garlic powder

Add the potatoes in the Ninja Foodi basket.

Cover with the crisping lid.

Set it to air crisp.

Cook at 400 degrees F for 16 minutes, flipping halfway through.

You can serve with vegan cheese sauce. Enjoy!

150. Garlic Chips

Servings: 2

Preparation Time: 70 Minutes

Calories: 156

Fat: 0.2 g

Protein: 4 g

Carbs: 35.4 g

Ingredients

2 potatoes, sliced into chips

Salt, to taste

4 garlic cloves

4 garlic cloves, minced

2 tbsp. vegan parmesan

Direction

Put the potatoes in a bowl of water

Stir in the salt.

Soak for 20 to 30 minutes.

Drain the potatoes and pat try.

Season with the garlic and vegan parmesan.

Arrange the chips on the Ninja Foodi basket.

Seal the crisping lid.

Set it to air crisp function.

Cook at 350 degrees for 10 minutes or until crispy.

Flip every 3 to 5 minutes.

You can serve with hot sauce or mayo. Enjoy!

151. Cauliflower Stir Fry

Servings: 4

Preparation Time: 40 Minutes

Calories: 93

Fat: 3 g

Protein: 4 g

Carbs: 12 g

Ingredients

1 head cauliflower, sliced into florets

3/4 cup white onion, sliced

5 garlic cloves, minced

1 1/2 tsp. tamari

1 tbsp. rice vinegar

1/2 tsp. coconut sugar

1 tbsp. hot sauce

Direction

Put the cauliflower in the Ninja Foodi basket.

Seal the crisping lid.

Select the air crisp setting.

Cook at 350 degrees F for 10 minutes.

Add the onion, stir and cook for additional 10 minutes.

Add the garlic, and cook for 5 minutes.

Mix the rest of the ingredients.

Pour over the cauliflower before serving.

You can garnish with chopped scallions. Enjoy!

152. Vegan Cheese Sticks

Servings: 3

Preparation Time: 8 Hours 40 Minutes

Calories: 116

Fat: 4.1 g

Protein: 12.7 g

Carbs: 9.7 g

Ingredients

1 block vegan mozzarella, sliced into strips

1 bag vegan chips

1 1/2 cups almond flour

2 cups vegan milk

1/4 cup nutritional yeast

Direction

Put the chips and nutritional yeast in the food processor.

Pulse until powdery.

Dip each cheese strip in the milk and cover with flour.

Dip into the milk again and coat with the powdered chips.

Place in the freezer for 8 hours.

Add the frozen cheese sticks to the Ninja Foodi basket.

Seal the crisping lid.

Set it to air crisp.

Cook at 380 degrees for 10 minutes.

You can serve with vegetable sticks. Enjoy!

153. Smoked Chickpeas

Servings: 3

Preparation Time: 45 Minutes

Calories: 423

Fat: 10.1 g

Protein: 20.8 g

Carbs: 65.2 g

Ingredients

15 oz. chickpeas, rinsed and drained

1 tbsp. sunflower oil

2 tbsp. smoked paprika

1/2 tsp. granulated garlic

1/2 tsp. ground cumin

1/4 tsp. granulated onion

Salt, to taste

Direction

Mix all the ingredients except the oil and chickpeas.

Put the chickpeas in the Ninja Foodi basket.

Seal the crisping lid.

Set it to air crisp function.

Cook at 390 degrees F for 15 minutes, shaking halfway through.

Put the chickpeas in the bowl of seasonings.

Put them back to the Ninja Foodi basket.

Cook at 360 degrees F for 3 minutes.

You can add cayenne pepper to make the dish spicier. Enjoy!

154. Fried Broccoli

Servings: 2

Preparation Time: 25 Minutes

Calories: 197

Fat: 14.5 g

Protein: 7.4 g

Carbs: 14.4 g

Ingredients

4 cups broccoli florets

2 tbsp. coconut oil

1 tbsp. nutritional yeast

Salt and pepper, to taste

Direction

Combine all the ingredients in a bowl.

Place the broccoli in the Ninja Foodi basket.

Seal the crisping lid.

Choose air crisp setting.

Cook at 370 degrees F for 5 minutes.

You can serve as side dish. Enjoy!

155. Garlic Pepper Potato Chips

Servings: 2

Preparation Time: 30 Minutes

Calories: 197

Fat: 14.5 g

Protein: 7.4 g

Carbs: 14.4 g

Ingredients

1 large potato, sliced into thin chips

Cooking spray

Salt and garlic powder, to taste

1 tsp. black pepper

Direction

Spray oil on the Ninja Foodi basket.

Season the potato with the salt, garlic powder and black pepper.

Place potato chips on the basket.

Seal the crisping lid.

Set it to air crisp.

Cook at 450 degrees F for 10 minutes or until golden and crispy.

You can serve with mayo dip. Enjoy!

156. Crispy Brussels Sprouts

Servings: 4

Preparation Time: 30 Minutes

Calories: 139

Fat: 5.4 g

Protein: 7.8 g

Carbs: 20.9 g

Ingredients

1 lb. Brussels sprouts

2 tbsp. olive oil

1/4 tsp. garlic powder

1/4 tsp. salt

Direction

Put the Brussels sprouts in a bowl.

Pour the olive oil into the bowl.

Season the sprouts with garlic powder and salt.

Put the sprouts on the basket.

Seal the crisping lid.

Set it to air crisp function.

Cook at 370 degrees F for 6 minutes, flipping halfway through.

You can serve as side dish. Enjoy!

157. Veggie Fritters

Servings: 6

Preparation Time: 45 Minutes

Calories: 171

Fat: 0.5 g

Protein: 5.8 g

Carbs: 35.7 g

Ingredients

3 tbsp. ground flaxseed mixed with 1/2 cup water

2 potatoes, shredded

2 cups frozen mixed veggies

1 cup frozen peas, thawed

1/2 cup onion, chopped

1/4 cup fresh cilantro, chopped

1/2 cup almond flour

Salt, to taste

Cooking spray

Direction

Combine all the ingredients in a bowl and then form patties.

Spray each patty with oil.

Transfer to the Ninja Foodi basket.

Set it to air crisp.

Close the crisping lid.

Cook at 360 degrees F for 15 minutes, flipping halfway through.

Transfer to a serving plate. Serve and enjoy!

158. Steamed Broccoli And Carrots With Lemon

Servings: 3

Preparation Time: 10 Minutes

Calories: 35

Fat: 0.3 g

Protein: 1.7 g

Carbs: 8.1 g

Ingredients

1 cup broccoli florets

1/2 cup carrots, julienned

2 tbsp. lemon juice

Salt and pepper, to taste

Direction

Place the Ninja Foodi Cook and Crisp reversible rack inside the ceramic pot.

Pour water into the pot.

Toss everything in a mixing bowl and combine.

Place the vegetables on the reversible rack.

Close the pressure lid and set the vent to SEAL.

Press the Steam button and adjust the cooking time to 10 minutes.

Do a quick pressure release. Serve and enjoy!

159. Crusty Sweet Potato Hash

Servings: 4

Preparation Time: 15 Minutes

Calories: 195

Fat: 6 g

Protein: 3.7 g

Carbs: 31.4 g

Ingredients

2 large sweet potatoes, cut into small cubes

2 slices bacon, cut into small pieces

2 tbsp. olive oil

1 tbsp. smoked paprika

2 tsp. salt

1 tsp. ground black pepper

1 tsp. dill weed

Direction

Place in the ceramic pot the Ninja Foodi Cook and Crisp basket.

Combine all ingredients in a bowl and give a good stir.

Form small patties using your hands.

Place the patties in the basket.

Close the crisping lid and press the Air Crisp button before pressing the START button.

Adjust the cooking time to 10 minutes.

Flip the patties halfway through the cooking time for even cooking. Serve and enjoy!

160. Cheesy Potato Gratin

Preparation Time: 10 minutes

Cooking Time: 30 minutes

Servings 6

Ingredients:

3 medium potatoes, sliced 1/8-inch thick

3 cups cheddar cheese, shredded

3/4 cup heavy cream

3/4 tsp garlic powder

1 tbsp butter

1/4 tsp pepper

1/2 tsp sea salt

Directions:

Spray 8-inch round pan with cooking spray.

Layer the sliced potatoes in prepared pan.

Season each layer with garlic powder, pepper, and salt then pour 1 tablespoon of heavy cream over potato layer and sprinkle thin layer of shredded cheese.

Layer sliced potatoes until you have 5 layers.

Top with remaining cream and cheese.

Pour 1 1/2 cups of water into the instant pot duo crisp then place the trivet in the pot.

Place pan on top of the trivet.

Seal the pot with pressure cooking lid and cook on pressure cook mode for 25 minutes.

Once done, release pressure using a quick release. Remove lid.

Seal the pot with air fryer lid and select broil mode for 5 minutes.

Once done then remove the pan from instant pot and let it cool for 10 minutes.

Serve and enjoy.

Nutrition:

Calories 371

Fat 26.3 g

Carbohydrates 18.2 g

Sugar 1.6 g

Protein 16.3 g

Cholesterol 85 mg

161. Crispy Mac & Cheese

Preparation Time: 10 minutes

Cooking Time: 9 minutes

Servings 6

Ingredients:

2 1/2 cups macaroni

1/4 tsp garlic powder

1 sleeve crackers, crushed

1/3 cup parmesan cheese, shredded

2 2/3 cups cheddar cheese, shredded

1/2 cup butter

1 cup heavy cream

2 cups vegetable stock

Pepper

Salt

Directions:

Add stock, heavy cream, 1/4 cup of butter, and macaroni in the instant pot duo crisp and stir well.

Seal the pot with pressure cooking lid and cook on high pressure for 4 minutes.

Once done, release pressure using a quick release. Remove lid.

Add 2 cups of shredded cheddar cheese and stir until cheese is melted.

Mix together remaining butter and crushed crackers.

Add remaining cheddar cheese, parmesan cheese, and crushed crackers on top of the macaroni mixture.

Seal the pot with air fryer lid and air fry for 5 minutes at 400 F.

Serve and enjoy.

Nutrition:

Calories 674

Fat 55 g

Carbohydrates 20 g

Sugar 3 g

Protein 20 g

Cholesterol 160 mg

162. Crispy Roasted Potatoes

Preparation Time: 10 minutes

Cooking Time: 16 minutes

Servings 4

Ingredients:

2 lbs baby potatoes, scrubbed and pierced with a fork

2 tbsp olive oil

1 cup vegetable broth

2 garlic cloves, peeled

Pepper

Salt

For seasoning:

1/8 tsp nutmeg

1/2 tsp sage

1/2 tsp thyme

1/2 tsp oregano

1 tsp rosemary

1/8 tsp pepper

Directions:

Add Baby potatoes, broth, and garlic into the instant pot duo crisp.

Seal the pot with pressure cooking lid and cook on pressure cook mode for 11 minutes.

Once done, release pressure using a quick release. Remove lid.

Drain out the broth and pat dry potatoes.

Add oil into the instant pot and set the pot on sauté mode.

Once the oil is hot then add potatoes and all seasonings and cook on sauté mode for 5 minutes or until potatoes are lightly brown.

Serve and enjoy.

Nutrition:

Calories 206

Fat 7.7 g

Carbohydrates 29.5 g

Sugar 0.2 g

Protein 7.2 g

Cholesterol 0 mg

163. Crispy Honey Carrots

Preparation Time: 10 minutes

Cooking Time: 10 minutes

Servings 2

Ingredients:

3 cups carrots, cut into 1/2-inch pieces

1 tbsp honey

1 tbsp olive oil

Pepper

Salt

Directions:

Add carrots in a mixing bowl then add honey, oil, pepper, and salt and toss to coat.

Transfer carrots into the instant pot duo crisp air fryer basket then place basket in the instant pot.

Seal the pot with air fryer lid and air fry carrots for 10 minutes at 400 F. Toss carrots after 5 minutes.

Serve and enjoy.

Nutrition:

Calories 160

Fat 7 g

Carbohydrates 24.9 g

Sugar 16.7 g

Protein 1.4 g

Cholesterol 0 mg

164. Perfect Mashed Potatoes

Preparation Time: 10 minutes

Cooking Time: 7 minutes

Servings 6

Ingredients:

3 lbs potatoes, peeled and cut into 1 1/2-inch pieces

1/4 cup half and half

1/4 cup butter

1 lb parsnips, cut into 1-inch pieces

Pepper

Salt

Directions:

Pour 2 cups of water into the instant pot.

Add potatoes and parsnips into the air fryer basket then place a basket in the instant pot.

Seal the pot with pressure cooking lid and select pressure cook for 7 minutes.

Once done, release pressure using a quick release. Remove lid.

Transfer potatoes and parsnips into the mixing bowl. Using masher mash until smooth.

Add half and half, butter, pepper, and salt and mix well.

Serve and enjoy.

Nutrition:

Calories 294

Fat 9.3 g

Carbohydrates 49.7 g

Sugar 6.3 g

Protein 5.1 g

Cholesterol 24 mg

165. Ranch Carrots

Preparation Time: 10 minutes

Cooking Time: 3 hours

Servings 4

Ingredients:

2 lbs carrots, cut into fries shape

1/4 cup butter

1 onion, diced

1 tbsp ranch seasoning

Pepper

Salt

Directions:

Add all ingredients into the inner pot of instant pot duo crisp. Stir well.

Seal the pot with pressure cooking lid and select slow cook mode and cook on high for 4 hours.

Serve and enjoy.

Nutrition:

Calories 213

Fat 11.5 g

Carbohydrates 24.9 g

Sugar 12.3 g

Protein 2.3 g

Cholesterol 31 mg

166. Creamy Sweet Potato Mash

Preparation Time: 10 minutes

Cooking Time: 4 hours

Servings 6

Ingredients:

4 lbs sweet potatoes, peel and diced

3/4 tsp curry powder

1 cup vegetable stock

2 tbsp butter

1/4 cup coconut milk

Pepper

Salt

Directions:

Add sweet potatoes and vegetable stock into the inner pot of instant pot duo crisp.

Seal the pot with pressure cooking lid and select slow cook mode and cook on low for 4 hours.

Mash sweet potatoes using masher until smooth.

Add butter, coconut milk, and curry powder and mix well.

Season with pepper and salt.

Serve and enjoy.

Nutrition:

Calories 416

Fat 6.8 g

Carbohydrates 85.2 g

Sugar 2 g

Protein 5 g

Cholesterol 10 mg

167. Delicious Fruit Salsa

Preparation Time: 10 minutes

Cooking Time: 2 hours

Servings 6

Ingredients:

1/2 red bell pepper, chopped

1/2 yellow bell pepper, chopped

1/2 green bell pepper, chopped

8 oz can pineapple tidbits

8 oz can peach, sliced

10 oz can oranges

3 tbsp cornstarch

3 tsp vinegar

1 tsp garlic, minced

1 medium onion, chopped

Directions:

Add all ingredients into the inner pot of instant pot duo crisp and stir well.

Seal the pot with pressure cooking lid and select slow cook mode and cook on high for 2 hours.

Stir and serve.

Nutrition:

Calories 101

Fat 0.2 g

Carbohydrates 24.3 g

Sugar 13.7 g

Protein 1.4 g

Cholesterol 0 mg

168. Easy Dill Carrots

Preparation Time: 10 minutes

Cooking Time: 2 hours

Servings 4

Ingredients:

1 lb carrots, cut round slices

1/2 tsp butter

3/4 tbsp fresh dill, minced

3 tbsp water

Directions:

Add all ingredients into the inner pot of instant pot duo crisp and stir well.

Seal the pot with pressure cooking lid and select slow cook mode and cook on low for 2 hours.

Stir and serve.

Nutrition:

Calories 52

Fat 0.5 g

Carbohydrates 11.5 g

Sugar 5.6 g

Protein 1.1 g

Cholesterol 1 mg

169. Tasty Ranch Potatoes

Preparation Time: 10 minutes

Cooking Time: 4 hours

Servings 4

Ingredients:

1 lb potatoes, diced

1/2 tsp onion powder

3/4 tsp garlic powder

1 tsp parsley, dried

1/4 cup butter, melted

1/4 tsp pepper

1/4 tsp dill, dried

1/2 tsp sea salt

Directions:

In a bowl, add 2 tbsp butter, potatoes, parsley, garlic powder, onion powder, sea salt, dill, and pepper. Toss well.

Transfer potato mixture to a foil piece and fold foil to cover potato mixture and place in the inner pot of instant pot duo crisp.

Seal the pot with pressure cooking lid and select slow cook mode and cook on low for 4 hours.

Open foil carefully and add remaining butter and mix well.

Serve and enjoy.

Nutrition:

Calories 183

Fat 11.6 g

Carbohydrates 18.6 g

Sugar 1.6 g

Protein 2.2 g

Cholesterol 31 mg

170. Healthy Summer Vegetables

Preparation Time: 10 minutes

Cooking Time: 4 hours

Servings 4

Ingredients:

1 1/2 cups zucchini, sliced

1 tsp butter

1/2 cup okra, diced

1/4 cup lemon juice

1 1/2 cups yellow squash, sliced

1 medium onion, sliced

1 tbsp thyme, minced

1/4 tsp pepper

1/4 tsp salt

Directions:

Add the onion in the inner pot of instant pot duo crisp then top with yellow squash, zucchini, pepper, lemon juice, thyme, and salt.

Seal the pot with pressure cooking lid and select slow cook mode and cook on low for 3 1/2 hours.

Add butter and okra and stir well.

Seal the pot again with pressure cooking lid and select slow cook mode and cook on high for 30 minutes more.

Serve and enjoy.

Nutrition:

Calories 45

Fat 1.3 g

Carbohydrates 7.8 g

Sugar 3.1 g

Protein 1.9 g

Cholesterol 3 mg

171. Stewed Okra

Preparation Time: 10 minutes

Cooking Time: 2 hours

Servings 4

Ingredients:

1 1/2 cups okra, diced

14 oz can tomato, crushed

1 tsp hot sauce

1 tsp garlic, minced

1 small onion, diced

Directions:

Add all ingredients into the inner pot of instant pot duo crisp and stir well.

Seal the pot with pressure cooking lid and select slow cook mode and cook on low for 2 hours.

Stir well and serve.

Nutrition:

Calories 44

Fat 0.1 g

Carbohydrates 9.7 g

Sugar 4.7 g

Protein 1.9 g

Cholesterol 0 mg

172. Roasted Vegetables

Preparation Time: 10 minutes

Cooking Time: 45 minutes

Servings 3

Ingredients:

4 carrots, peeled and cut into 3-inch pieces

5 potatoes, quartered

3 shallots, peeled and cut into half

1 tbsp olive oil

1/4 tsp garlic powder

Pepper

Salt

Directions:

Add carrots, potatoes, and shallots to the mixing bowl. Add oil, garlic powder, pepper, and salt over vegetables and toss well.

Line instant pot duo crisp air fryer basket with parchment paper or foil.

Add vegetables into the air fryer basket then place basket in the pot.

Seal the pot with air fryer lid and select roast mode and cook at 400 F for 45 minutes.

Serve and enjoy.

Nutrition:

Calories 326

Fat 5 g

Carbohydrates 65.6 g

Sugar 8.1 g

Protein 6.9 g

Cholesterol 0 mg

173. Delicious Potato Wedges

Preparation Time: 10 minutes

Cooking Time: 17 minutes

Servings 6

Ingredients:

1 1/2 lbs russet potatoes, cut into wedges

3/4 tsp garlic powder

1/2 tsp onion powder

1/4 cup olive oil

1 cup vegetable broth

1 tsp paprika

1/4 tsp pepper

1 tsp sea salt

Directions:

Add oil into the inner pot of instant pot duo crisp and set pot on sauté mode.

Add potatoes and sauté for 3-5 minutes.

Add remaining ingredients and stir well.

Seal the pot with pressure cooking lid and cook on high pressure for 7 minutes.

Once done, release pressure using a quick release. Remove lid.

Remove potato wedges from the pot and clean the pot.

Add potato wedges into the air fryer basket and place basket in the pot.

Seal the pot with air fryer lid and select broil and cook for 5 minutes.

Serve and enjoy.

Nutrition:

Calories 160

Fat 8.8 g

Carbohydrates 18.6 g

Sugar 1.6 g

Protein 2.9 g

Cholesterol 0 mg

174. Crispy Ranch Potatoes

Preparation Time: 10 minutes

Cooking Time: 10 minutes

Servings 2

Ingredients:

1/2 lb potatoes, cut into 1-inch pieces

1 tbsp ranch seasoning

1/2 tbsp olive oil

Directions:

Add all ingredients into the bowl and toss well.

Transfer potato into the instant pot air fryer basket and place basket in the pot.

Seal the pot with air fryer lid and select air fry mode and cook at 375 F for 10 minutes.

Serve and enjoy.

Nutrition:

Calories 123

Fat 3.6 g

Carbohydrates 17.8 g

Sugar 1.3 g

Protein 1.9 g

Cholesterol 0 mg

175. Healthy Roasted Vegetables

Preparation Time: 10 minutes

Cooking Time: 45 minutes

Servings 4

Ingredients:

2 potatoes, cut into chunks

3 medium carrots, peeled and cut into chunks

1 small rutabaga, peeled and cut into chunks

2 parsnips, peeled and cut into chunks

1/4 cup olive oil

Pepper

Salt

Directions:

In a large bowl, toss vegetable with oil.

Transfer vegetables into the instant pot air fryer basket and season with pepper and salt.

Place air fryer basket in the pot.

Seal the pot with air fryer lid and select roast mode and cook at 400 F for 35-45 minutes.

Nutrition:

Calories 267

Fat 13 g

Carbohydrates 37.1 g

Sugar 9.4 g

Protein 3.6 g

Cholesterol 0 mg

176. Pineapple Salsa

Preparation Time: 10 minutes

Cooking Time: 8 minutes

Servings 2

Ingredients:

1 cup pineapple, diced

1/3 cup cilantro, chopped

1 cup tomatoes, diced

1 cup peppers, diced

4 tbsp lime juice

1/4 cup onion, minced

Pepper

Salt

Directions:

Add all ingredients into the inner pot of instant pot duo crisp and stir well.

Seal the pot with pressure cooking lid and cook on high for 8 minutes.

Once done, release pressure using a quick release. Remove lid.

Stir and serve.

Nutrition:

Calories 137

Fat 1 g

Carbohydrates 35.6 g

Sugar 12.7 g

Protein 3.9 g

Cholesterol 0 mg

177. Banana Buckwheat Porridge

Preparation Time: 10 minutes

Cooking Time: 6 minutes

Servings 4

Ingredients:

1 cup raw buckwheat grouts, rinsed

1/4 cup raisins

1 banana, sliced

3 cups almond milk

1/2 tsp vanilla

1 tsp cinnamon

Directions:

Add all ingredients into the inner pot of instant pot duo crisp and stir well.

Seal the pot with pressure cooking lid and cook on high for 6 minutes.

Once done, allow to release pressure naturally. Remove lid.

Serve and enjoy.

Nutrition:

Calories 571

Fat 44 g

Carbohydrates 45.6 g

Sugar 15.8 g

Protein 8.5 g

Cholesterol 0 mg

178. Banana Oatmeal

Preparation Time: 10 minutes

Cooking Time: 5 minutes

Servings 2

Ingredients:

1 cup oatmeal

1 banana, sliced

1 cup of water

1 cup almond milk

1 tbsp maple syrup

1 1/2 tsp cinnamon

Directions:

Spray instant pot inner pot with cooking spray.

Add water, oatmeal, and almond milk and stir well.

Add maple syrup, cinnamon, and banana and stir well.

Seal the pot with pressure cooking lid and cook on high for 5 minutes.

Once done, allow to release pressure naturally. Remove lid.

Stir and serve.

Nutrition:

Calories 514

Fat 31.5 g

Carbohydrates 55.9 g

Sugar 17.6 g

Protein 8.8 g

Cholesterol 0 mg

179. Smooth Mashed Potatoes

Preparation Time: 10 minutes

Cooking Time: 25 minutes

Servings 4

Ingredients:

4 large potatoes, peeled and cubed

1 fresh sprig rosemary

2 garlic cloves

1 cup vegetable broth

1/4 cup almond milk

2 tbsp olive oil

Directions:

Add potatoes, rosemary, garlic, and broth into the inner pot of instant pot duo crisp and stir well.

Seal the pot with pressure cooking lid and cook on high for 25 minutes.

Once done, release pressure using a quick release. Remove lid.

Drain potatoes well and transfer to the large bowl. Remove rosemary sprig.

Add oil and almond milk and using potato masher mash the potatoes until smooth.

Serve warm and enjoy.

Nutrition:

Calories 364

Fat 11.4 g

Carbohydrates 60.1 g

Sugar 4.9 g

Protein 7.9 g

Cholesterol 0 mg

180. Delicious Chickpea Hummus

Preparation Time: 10 minutes

Cooking Time: 45 minutes

Servings 10

Ingredients:

1 cup chickpeas, dried

3 garlic cloves, minced

3 cups vegetable broth

1 tbsp fresh lemon juice

2 tbsp olive oil

1 tsp salt

Directions:

Add broth, chickpeas, and salt into the inner pot of instant pot duo crisp.

Seal the pot with pressure cooking lid and high for 45 minutes.

Once done, release pressure using a quick release. Remove lid.

Drain chickpeas well and transfer to the food processor along with remaining ingredients and process until smooth.

Serve and enjoy.

Nutrition:

Calories 110

Fat 4.4 g

Carbohydrates 12.7 g

Sugar 2.4 g

Protein 5.4 g

Cholesterol 0 mg

181. Herb Lentil Rice

Preparation Time: 10 minutes

Cooking Time: 25 minutes

Servings 4

Ingredients:

1 1/2 cups brown rice, uncooked

1 cup brown lentils, dried

3 1/2 cups water

1 tsp garlic cloves, minced

1/2 cup onion, chopped

1 tbsp thyme, dried

1 fresh rosemary sprig

1 cup potato, peeled and diced

1 tbsp olive oil

Pepper

Salt

Directions:

Add oil into the inner pot of instant pot duo crisp and set pot on sauté mode.

Add onion and sauté for 5 minutes. Add garlic and sauté for a minute.

Add remaining ingredients and stir well.

Seal the pot with pressure cooking lid and cook on high for 20 minutes.

Once done, allow to release pressure naturally. Remove lid.

Stir well and serve.

Nutrition:

Calories 352

Fat 5.8 g

Carbohydrates 66.2 g

Sugar 0.8 g

Protein 8.8 g

Cholesterol 0 mg

Chapter 7 Dinner Recipes

182. Easy Cilantro Lime Rice

Preparation Time: 10 minutes

Cooking Time: 12 minutes

Servings 6

Ingredients:

2 cups white rice, long grain

2 tbsp olive oil

3/4 cup water

14 oz vegetable broth

3/4 cup fresh cilantro, chopped

2 1/2 tbsp fresh lime juice

1/2 tsp salt

Directions:

Add rice, 2 tablespoon lime juice, oil, water, and broth in the inner pot of instant pot duo crisp and stir well.

Seal the pot with pressure cooking lid and cook on high for 12 minutes.

Once done, release pressure using a quick release. Remove lid.

Fluff the rice using a fork and transfer to the large bowl.

Add remaining lime juice, salt, and cilantro and stir well.

Serve and enjoy.

Nutrition:

Calories 281

Fat 5.5 g

Carbohydrates 51.2 g

Sugar 0.6 g

Protein 5.9 g

Cholesterol 0 mg

183. Spicy Rice

Preparation Time: 10 minutes

Cooking Time: 22 minutes

Servings 6

Ingredients:

2 cups brown rice, uncooked

1/2 tsp onion powder

2 tbsp tomato paste

1 tbsp cumin

2 tbsp chili powder

1/2 tsp garlic powder

2 cups vegetable broth

1 tsp salt

Directions:

Add water and rice into the inner pot of instant pot duo crisp.

Seal the pot with pressure cooking lid and cook on high for 22 minutes.

Once done, release pressure using a quick release. Remove lid.

Add remaining ingredients and stir well.

Serve and enjoy.

Nutrition:

Calories 259

Fat 2.8 g

Carbohydrates 51.7 g

Sugar 1.2 g

Protein 7.2 g

Cholesterol 0 mg

184. Refried Pinto Beans

Preparation Time: 10 minutes

Cooking Time: 35 minutes

Servings 8

Ingredients:

2 cups pinto beans, dried and rinsed

4 cups vegetable broth

1 jalapeno, minced

1 tbsp garlic, minced

1 onion, chopped

1 tsp ground cumin

1 1/2 tsp oregano

4 cups of water

1 tbsp olive oil

1/2 tsp pepper

1 tsp salt

Directions:

Add oil into the inner pot of instant pot duo crisp and set pot on sauté mode.

Add jalapeno, garlic, and onion and sauté until softened.

Add beans, seasoning, water, and broth. Stir well.

Seal the pot with pressure cooking lid and cook on high for 30 minutes.

Once done, allow to release pressure naturally. Remove lid.

Mash beans using potato mashed until desired consistency get.

Serve and enjoy.

Nutrition:

Calories 211

Fat 3.1 g

Carbohydrates 32.8 g

Sugar 2 g

Protein 13.1 g

Cholesterol 0 mg

185. Sweetcorn Risotto

Preparation Time: 10 minutes

Cooking Time: 13 minutes

Servings 4

Ingredients:

1 cup Arborio rice

1/2 cup sweet corn

1 tsp mix herbs

3 cups vegetable stock

1 tbsp olive oil

1 tsp garlic, minced

1/2 cup peas

1 red pepper, diced

1 large onion, chopped

1/4 pepper

1/2 tsp salt

Directions:

Add oil into the inner pot of instant pot duo crisp and set pot on sauté mode.

Add onion and garlic and sauté for 5 minutes.

Add rice and stir to combine.

Add remaining ingredients and stir well.

Seal the pot with pressure cooking lid and cook on high for 8 minutes.

Once done, release pressure using a quick release. Remove lid.

Serve and enjoy.

Nutrition:

Calories 269

Fat 4.8 g

Carbohydrates 50.8 g

Sugar 5.3 g

Protein 6.2 g

Cholesterol 0 mg

186. Sweet Carrots

Preparation Time: 10 minutes

Cooking Time: 3 minutes

Servings 8

Ingredients:

2 lbs carrots, peeled and sliced thickly

3 tbsp raisins

1 tbsp maple syrup

1 tbsp butter

1 cup of water

Pepper

Salt

Directions:

Add water, carrots, and raisins in the inner pot of instant pot duo crisp.

Seal the pot with pressure cooking lid and cook on high for 3 minutes.

Once done, release pressure using a quick release. Remove lid.

Drain carrots and transfer to the mixing bowl.

Add butter and maple syrup over carrots and toss well. Season with pepper and salt.

Serve and enjoy.

Nutrition:

Calories 76

Fat 1.5 g

Carbohydrates 15.5 g

Sugar 9.1 g

Protein 1.1 g

Cholesterol 4 mg

187. Spicy Rice

Preparation Time: 10 minutes

Cooking Time: 3 minutes

Servings 2

Ingredients:

1 cup rice, long grain

1/4 cup green hot sauce

1/2 cup fresh cilantro, chopped

1/2 avocado flesh

1 1/4 cup vegetable broth

Pepper

Salt

Directions:

Add broth and rice in the inner pot of instant pot duo crisp and stir well.

Seal the pot with pressure cooking lid and cook on high for 3 minutes.

Once done, allow to release pressure naturally. Remove lid.

Fluff the rice using a fork.

Add green sauce, avocado and cilantro in a blender and blend until smooth.

Pour blended mixture into the rice and stir well to combine. Season with pepper and salt.

Serve and enjoy.

Nutrition:

Calories 375

Fat 2.6 g

Carbohydrates 75.5 g

Sugar 0.6 g

Protein 10 g

Cholesterol 0 mg

188. Indian Potato Curry

Preparation Time: 10 minutes

Cooking Time: 7 minutes

Servings 4

Ingredients:

2 medium potatoes, peeled and chopped

1/2 tsp garam masala

1 Serrano, minced

1/2 cup onion masala

1 tsp cumin seeds

1 1/2 cups water

2 cups fresh peas

2 tbsp olive oil

1/4 tsp pepper

1 tsp salt

Directions:

Add oil into the inner pot of instant pot duo crisp and set pot on sauté mode.

Add Serrano pepper and cumin seeds and sauté for 1-2 minutes.

Add remaining ingredients and stir well.

Seal the pot with pressure cooking lid and cook on high for 5 minutes.

Once done, release pressure using a quick release. Remove lid.

Serve and enjoy.

Nutrition:

Calories 244

Fat 9.5 g

Carbohydrates 33.4 g

Sugar 6.2 g

Protein 7.7 g

Cholesterol 2 mg

189. Veggie Quinoa

Preparation Time: 10 minutes

Cooking Time: 7 minutes

Servings 4

Ingredients:

1 1/2 cups quinoa, rinsed and drained

1 carrot, chopped

1 cup green beans, chopped

1 potato, cubed

1 tomato, chopped

1 small onion, chopped

2 tsp ginger paste

1 garlic clove, minced

1/4 cup cilantro, chopped

1 1/2 cups water

1/4 cup coconut milk

1 tsp garam masala

1/2 tsp chili powder

1/2 tsp black pepper

1/4 tsp turmeric

1 bay leaf

4 cloves

1 tsp cumin seeds

2-star anise

2 tbsp olive oil

Salt

Directions:

Add oil into the inner pot of instant pot duo crisp and set pot on sauté mode.

Add cumin seeds, cloves, and star anise and sauté for 30 seconds. Add ginger and garlic and sauté for 1 minute.

Add tomatoes, onions, and dry spices and sauté for 1-2 minutes.

Add all the vegetables, salt, and coconut milk, water, and quinoa. Stir well.

Seal the pot with pressure cooking lid and cook on high for 4 minutes.

Once done, allow to release pressure naturally for 10 minutes then release remaining pressure using a quick release. Remove lid.

Serve and enjoy.

Nutrition:

Calories 404

Fat 15.2 g

Carbohydrates 58 g

Sugar 3.2 g

Protein 11.8 g

Cholesterol 0 mg

190. Healthy Quinoa Black Bean Chili

Preparation Time: 10 minutes

Cooking Time: 12 minutes

Servings 6

Ingredients:

1/2 cup quinoa, rinsed and drained

14 oz can black beans, rinsed and drained

14 oz can tomato, diced

2 tbsp tomato paste

4 cups vegetable broth

2 celery stalks, diced

1 tsp garlic, minced

1 onion, chopped

1 tsp chili powder

1 tsp ground coriander

2 tsp ground cumin

2 tsp paprika

3 sweet potatoes, peeled and diced

1 bell pepper, diced

1 tsp salt

Directions:

Add all ingredients into the inner pot of instant pot duo crisp and stir well.

Seal the pot with pressure cooking lid and cook on high for 12 minutes.

Once done, release pressure using a quick release. Remove lid.

Stir and serve.

Nutrition:

Calories 267

Fat 2.6 g

Carbohydrates 51.2 g

Sugar 6.2 g

Protein 11.5 g

Cholesterol 0 mg

191. Delicious Pigeon Pea

Preparation Time: 10 minutes

Cooking Time: 7 minutes

Servings 4

Ingredients:

1 cup split pigeon pea, rinsed and drained

1 tbsp ginger, chopped

1 green chili, sliced

1/4 tsp cumin seeds

1 tbsp olive oil

2 cups spinach

1/2 tsp garam masala

3 cups of water

1 large tomato, chopped

1 tbsp garlic, chopped

Spices:

1/4 tsp turmeric

1/2 tsp chili powder

1 tsp salt

Directions:

Add oil into the inner pot of instant pot duo crisp and set pot on sauté mode.

Add cumin seeds, garlic, ginger, and green chili and sauté for 30 seconds.

Add tomatoes and spices and sauté for 1 minute.

Add lentils and water. Stir well.

Seal the pot with pressure cooking lid and cook on high for 3 minutes.

Once done, release pressure using a quick release. Remove lid.

Set pot on sauté mode. Add spinach and garam masala and stir until spinach is wilted.

Serve and enjoy.

Nutrition:

Calories 97

Fat 4.3 g

Carbohydrates 12.2 g

Sugar 1.6 g

Protein 3.5 g

Cholesterol 0 mg

192. Flavorful Mushroom Rice

Preparation Time: 10 minutes

Cooking Time: 10 minutes

Servings 4

Ingredients:

2 cups rice, soak for 30 minutes and drained

1/2-inch cinnamon stick

2 tbsp vegetable oil

1/2 tsp caraway seed

15 oz mushrooms, sliced

2 tbsp cashews

1/4 cup coconut milk

4 cloves

2 cups of water

1/2 tsp garam masala

1 tsp chili powder

1/2 tsp turmeric

4 green cardamom

2-star anise

1 bay leaf

3 garlic cloves

1 tbsp ginger, minced

2 tbsp green chilies

1 onion, chopped

Salt

Directions:

Add oil into the inner pot of instant pot duo crisp and set pot on sauté mode.

Add cashews and sauté for a minute.

Add caraway seeds, green chilies, garlic, ginger, all dry spices and sauté for 1-2 minutes.

Add onion and cook for 2 minutes.

Add remaining ingredients and stir everything well.

Seal the pot with pressure cooking lid and cook on high for 4 minutes.

Once done, allow to release pressure naturally for 10 minutes then release remaining pressure using a quick release. Remove lid.

Stir and serve.

Nutrition:

Calories 530

Fat 14.3 g

Carbohydrates 90.5 g

Sugar 4.4 g

Protein 12.6 g

Cholesterol 0 mg

193. Rice Lentil Porridge

Preparation Time: 10 minutes

Cooking Time: 21 minutes

Servings 4

Ingredients:

1/2 cup yellow lentils, soaked for 15 minutes and drained

1 cup rice, soaked for 15 minutes and drained

6 cups vegetable stock

1 bay leaf

1 tsp turmeric

1 1/2 tsp cumin seeds

2 tbsp olive oil

1 1/2 tsp salt

Directions:

Add oil into the inner pot of instant pot duo crisp and set pot on sauté mode.

Add cumin seeds and bay leaf and sauté for 30 seconds.

Add lentils, turmeric, rice, salt, and stock. Stir well.

Seal the pot with pressure cooking lid and cook on high for minutes.

Once done, allow to release pressure naturally for 10 minutes then release remaining pressure using a quick release. Remove lid.

Stir and serve.

Nutrition:

Calories 320

Fat 7.9 g

Carbohydrates 51.9 g

Sugar 1.2 g

Protein 10.1 g

Cholesterol 0 mg

194. Wheat Berry Pilaf

Preparation Time: 10 minutes

Cooking Time: 35 minutes

Servings 6

Ingredients:

1 1/2 cups wheat berries, rinsed and drained

1/2 cup onion, minced

1 tsp coriander seeds

2 tsp cumin seeds

1 tbsp olive oil

3 cups of water

1 1/2 tsp turmeric

1 tbsp garlic, minced

Salt

Directions:

Add oil into the inner pot of instant pot duo crisp and set pot on sauté mode.

Add onion and cook until softened.

Add turmeric, garlic, coriander, and cumin and sauté for 2 minutes.

Add wheat berries and sauté for 2 minutes.

Add water and stir everything well.

Seal the pot with pressure cooking lid and cook on high for 30 minutes.

Once done, allow to release pressure naturally. Remove lid.

Stir well and serve.

Nutrition:

Calories 84

Fat 2.9 g

Carbohydrates 13.5 g

Sugar 0.5 g

Protein 2.4 g

Cholesterol 0 mg

195. Spicy Tomato Chutney

Preparation Time: 10 minutes

Cooking Time: 6 minutes

Servings 4

Ingredients:

4 green tomatoes, chopped

1/2 tsp mustard seeds

1 tbsp brown sugar

2 jalapeno pepper, chopped

1/2 tsp turmeric

1 tbsp olive oil

1 tsp salt

Directions:

Add oil into the inner pot of instant pot duo crisp and set pot on sauté mode.

Once the oil is hot then add mustard seeds and let them pop.

Add remaining ingredients and stir well.

Seal the pot with pressure cooking lid and cook on high for 5 minutes.

Once done, release pressure using a quick release. Remove lid.

Mash tomatoes mixture using a potato masher until getting the desired consistency.

Serve and enjoy.

Nutrition:

Calories 66

Fat 3.9 g

Carbohydrates 7.7 g

Sugar 5.7 g

Protein 1.3 g

Cholesterol 0 mg

196. Roasted Beans

Preparation Time: 10 minutes

Cooking Time: 30 minutes

Servings 4

Ingredients:

1 lb green beans

1/2 tsp onion powder

2 tbsp olive oil

3/4 tsp garlic powder

1/2 tsp pepper

1/2 tsp salt

Directions:

In a large bowl, add all ingredients and toss well.

Arrange green beans into the instant pot air fryer basket and place basket in the pot.

Seal the pot with air fryer lid and select bake mode and cook at 400 F for 25-30 minutes.

Serve and enjoy.

Nutrition:

Calories 99

Fat 7.2 g

Carbohydrates 8.9 g

Sugar 1.8 g

Protein 2.2 g

Cholesterol 0 mg

197. Parmesan Zucchini & Eggplant

Preparation Time: 10 minutes

Cooking Time: 35 minutes

Servings 6

Ingredients:

1 eggplant, sliced

1 tbsp olive oil

1 tbsp garlic, minced

1 cup cherry tomatoes, halved

3 medium zucchinis, sliced

1/4 cup basil, chopped

3 oz Parmesan cheese, grated

1/4 cup parsley, chopped

1/4 tsp pepper

1/4 tsp salt

Directions:

Line instant pot air fryer basket with parchment paper or foil.

In a mixing bowl, add cherry tomatoes, eggplant, zucchini, olive oil, garlic, cheese, basil, pepper, and salt toss well.

Transfer vegetable mixture into the air fryer basket and place basket in the pot.

Seal the pot with air fryer basket and select bake mode and cook at 350 F for 35 minutes.

Garnish with parsley and serve.

Nutrition:

Calories 109

Fat 5.8 g

Carbohydrates 10.2 g

Sugar 4.8 g

Protein 7 g

Cholesterol 10 mg

198. Roasted Vegetables

Preparation Time: 10 minutes

Cooking Time: 30 minutes

Servings 4

Ingredients:

8 oz carrots, cut into wedges

2 shallots, quartered

8 oz baby potatoes, wash and cut in half

8 oz Brussels sprouts, halved

2 tbsp balsamic vinegar

1 tbsp honey

3 tbsp olive oil

1/2 tsp pepper

3/4 tsp salt

Directions:

Spray baking instant pot air fryer basket with cooking spray.

In a large bowl, add shallots, potatoes, carrots, Brussels sprouts, olive oil, honey, vinegar, pepper and salt. Toss well.

Transfer vegetables into the air fryer basket and place basket in the pot.

Seal the pot with air fryer lid and select roast mode and cook at 400 F for 30 minutes.

Serve and enjoy.

Nutrition:

Calories 192

Fat 10.8 g

Carbohydrates 23.2 g

Sugar 8.4 g

Protein 4 g

Cholesterol 0 mg

199. Healthy Pumpkin Porridge

Preparation Time: 10 minutes

Cooking Time: 3 minutes

Servings 2

Ingredients:

1/2 cup pumpkin puree

3/4 tsp pumpkin pie spice

1/2 cup almond milk

1 1/4 cups water

1 tbsp brown sugar

1 cup quick oats

Directions:

Add all ingredients into the inner pot of instant pot duo crisp and stir well.

Seal the pot with pressure cooking lid and cook on high for 3 minutes.

Once done, allow to release pressure naturally. Remove lid.

Stir and serve warm.

Nutrition:

Calories 333

Fat 17.2 g

Carbohydrates 40.8 g

Sugar 8.9 g

Protein 7.5 g

Cholesterol 0 mg

200. Easy Apple Cinnamon Oatmeal

Preparation Time: 10 minutes

Cooking Time: 3 minutes

Servings 2

Ingredients:

1 cup quick oats

3 cups of water

3/4 tsp cinnamon

2 medium apples, chopped

Directions:

Add water and oats into the inner pot of instant pot duo crisp.

Seal the pot with pressure cooking lid and cook on high for 3 minutes.

Once done, allow to release pressure naturally. Remove lid.

Just before serving add apple and cinnamon.

Stir and serve.

Nutrition:

Calories 273

Fat 3.1 g

Carbohydrates 59.2 g

Sugar 23.6 g

Protein 6 g

Cholesterol 0 mg

201. Spinach Risotto

Preparation Time: 10 minutes

Cooking Time: 10 minutes

Servings 4

Ingredients:

1 1/2 cups Arborio rice

8 oz mushrooms, sliced

1 1/2 cups butternut squash, peeled and diced

1/2 cup dry white wine

3 1/2 cups vegetable broth

1 bell pepper, diced

1 tbsp garlic, minced

1 onion, chopped

3 cups spinach, chopped

1/4 tsp oregano

1/2 tsp coriander

1 tbsp olive oil

1 tsp pepper

1 tsp salt

Directions:

Add oil into the inner pot of instant pot duo crisp and set pot on sauté mode.

Add squash, bell pepper, garlic, and onion and sauté for 5 minutes.

Add remaining ingredients except spinach and stir well.

Seal the pot with pressure cooking lid and cook on high for 5 minutes.

Once done, release pressure using a quick release. Remove lid.

Add spinach and stir well and let it sit for 5 minutes.

Stir well and serve.

Nutrition:

Calories 411

Fat 5.5 g

Carbohydrates 73 g

Sugar 5.8 g

Protein 12.7 g

Cholesterol 0 mg

202. Chickpea Stew

Preparation Time: 10 minutes

Cooking Time: 25 minutes

Servings 6

Ingredients:

28 oz cans chickpeas, rinsed and drained

1/2 tsp ground cumin

1 tsp smoked paprika

2 large onion, chopped

2 tbsp olive oil

24 oz can tomato

1/4 cup dates, pitted and chopped

1/4 tsp allspice

1/2 tsp sea salt

Directions:

Add oil into the inner pot of instant pot duo crisp and set pot on sauté mode.

Add onion, allspice, cumin, paprika and salt and sauté for 5 minutes.

Add remaining ingredients and stir well.

Seal the pot with pressure cooking lid and cook on high for 20 minutes.

Once done, allow to release pressure naturally. Remove lid.

Stir and serve.

Nutrition:

Calories 264

Fat 6.4 g

Carbohydrates 46.2 g

Sugar 10.7 g

Protein 8.4 g

Cholesterol 0 mg

203. Quick Veggie Pasta

Preparation Time: 10 minutes

Cooking Time: 4 minutes

Servings 4

Ingredients:

1/2 lb pasta, uncooked

1/4 green onion, sliced

1/4 tsp red chili flakes

1 tsp ground ginger

1 tbsp garlic, minced

3 tbsp coconut amino

2 cups vegetable broth

1 1/2 cups baby spinach, chopped

1 cup frozen peas

8 oz mushrooms, sliced

2 carrots, peeled and chopped

1/4 tsp pepper

1 tsp salt

Directions:

Add all ingredients except spinach into the inner pot of instant pot duo crisp and stir well.

Seal the pot with pressure cooking lid and cook on high for 4 minutes.

Once done, allow to release pressure naturally. Remove lid.

Add spinach and stir well and let it sit for 5 minutes.

Serve and enjoy.

Nutrition:

Calories 258

Fat 2.3 g

Carbohydrates 45.9 g

Sugar 4.8 g

Protein 13.4 g

Cholesterol 41 mg

204. Baked Beans

Preparation Time: 10 minutes

Cooking Time: 40 minutes

Servings 4

Ingredients:

1 cup navy beans, dry, soaked overnight and drained

2 tbsp tomato paste

1/2 tbsp vinegar

1/2 tbsp Worcestershire sauce

1/2 tsp mustard

1 onion, chopped

1 tbsp olive oil

1/2 cup water

1/2 cup vegetable stock

1 1/2 tbsp molasses

2 tbsp brown sugar

1/2 tsp pepper

1/2 tsp sea salt

Directions:

Add oil into the inner pot of instant pot duo crisp and set pot on sauté mode.

Add onion and sauté for 3 minutes.

Add remaining ingredients and stir to combine.

Seal the pot with pressure cooking lid and cook on high for 40 minutes.

Once done, release pressure using a quick release. Remove lid.

Stir well and serve.

Nutrition:

Calories 267

Fat 4.5 g

Carbohydrates 46.5 g

Sugar 13.2 g

Protein 12.5 g

Cholesterol 0 mg

205. Easy Lentil Tacos

Preparation Time: 10 minutes

Cooking Time: 15 minutes

Servings 4

Ingredients:

2 cups brown lentils

1 tsp chili powder

1/2 tsp onion powder

1/2 cup tomato paste

4 cups vegetable broth

1/2 tsp ground cumin

1/2 tsp garlic powder

1 tsp salt

Directions:

Add all ingredients into the inner pot of instant pot duo crisp and stir well.

Seal the pot with pressure cooking lid and cook on high for 15 minutes.

Once done, release pressure using a quick release. Remove lid.

Stir well and serve.

Nutrition:

Calories 108

Fat 1.9 g

Carbohydrates 13 g

Sugar 5.5 g

Protein 9 g

Cholesterol 0 mg

206. Rice Black Bean Burritos

Preparation Time: 10 minutes

Cooking Time: 24 minutes

Servings 4

Ingredients:

1 cup black beans, dry, soaked overnight and drained

2 cups brown rice

1 tsp paprika

1 tbsp ground cumin

1 onion, chopped

1 tbsp chili powder

4 1/2 vegetable broth

1 cup tomato puree

1 tsp olive oil

1 tsp garlic, minced

Directions:

Add oil into the inner pot of instant pot duo crisp and set pot on sauté mode.

Add garlic and onion and sauté for 2 minutes.

Add 2 cups broth and rice. Stir well.

Seal the pot with pressure cooking lid and cook on high for 12 minutes.

Once done, release pressure using a quick release. Remove lid.

Add beans, remaining broth, chili powder, cumin, tomato puree, and paprika. Stir well.

Seal the pot again with pressure cooking lid and cook on high for 10 minutes.

Once done, allow to release pressure naturally. Remove lid.

Serve in a tortilla.

Nutrition:

Calories 618

Fat 5.3 g

Carbohydrates 124.3 g

Sugar 5.5 g

Protein 20.7 g

Cholesterol 0 mg

207. Veggie Risotto

Preparation Time: 10 minutes

Cooking Time: 13 minutes

Servings 4

Ingredients:

1 cup Arborio rice

1/2 cup peas

1 red pepper, diced

1 onion, chopped

1 tsp dried mix herbs

3 cups vegetable stock

1 tbsp olive oil

1 tsp garlic, minced

1/2 cup corn

1/4 pepper

1/2 tsp salt

Directions:

Add oil into the inner pot of instant pot duo crisp and set pot on sauté mode.

Add onion and garlic and sauté for 5 minutes.

Add rice and stir well. Add remaining ingredients and stir well.

Seal the pot with pressure cooking lid and cook on high for 8 minutes.

Once done, release pressure using a quick release. Remove lid.

Stir and serve.

Nutrition:

Calories 288

Fat 4.2 g

Carbohydrates 56 g

Sugar 5.4 g

Protein 6.7 g

Cholesterol 0 mg

208. Tasty Pumpkin Risotto

Preparation Time: 10 minutes

Cooking Time: 15 minutes

Servings 8

Ingredients:

3 cups pumpkin, diced

1 cup cream cheese

1 tsp sage, dried

3 tbsp olive oil

4 cups vegetable broth

2 tbsp white wine

1 onion, chopped

1 tsp garlic, minced

Directions:

Add oil, garlic, and onion into the inner pot of instant pot duo crisp and set pot on sauté mode. Sauté onion until soften.

Add pumpkin and sauté for a minute.

Add white wine, sage, rice, and broth and stir well.

Seal the pot with pressure cooking lid and cook on high for 10 minutes.

Once done, allow to release pressure naturally. Remove lid.

Add cream cheese and stir well.

Serve and enjoy.

Nutrition:

Calories 377

Fat 16.6 g

Carbohydrates 48 g

Sugar 4.1 g

Protein 9 g

Cholesterol 32 mg

209. Roasted Broccoli With Cashews

Preparation Time: 10 minutes

Cooking Time: 15 minutes

Servings 2

Ingredients:

3 cups broccoli florets

1/2 tbsp coconut amino

1/4 cup cashews, roasted

1 tbsp olive oil

1/2 tsp salt

Directions:

In a bowl, add broccoli, salt, and oil. Toss well.

Place broccoli into the instant pot air fryer basket and place basket into the pot.

Seal the pot with air fryer lid and select bake mode and cook at 375 F for 15 minutes.

In a large bowl, add roasted broccoli, cashews and coconut amino and toss well.

Serve and enjoy.

Nutrition:

Calories 209

Fat 15.4 g

Carbohydrates 15.4 g

Sugar 3.2 g

Protein 6.4 g

Cholesterol 0 mg

210. Vegan Balls

Servings: 6

Preparation Time: 20 minutes

Cooking Time: 20 minutes

Ingredients:

1/2 cup desiccated coconut

1 cup gluten-free oats

1 teaspoon chives

1 teaspoon mixed spice

1 teaspoon paprika

100 grams sweet potato

2 teaspoon garlic puree

2 teaspoon oregano

200 grams cauliflower

70 grams carrot

90 grams parsnips

Salt and pepper

Directions:

Put the raw vegetables into the food processor and process until the mixture resembles breadcrumbs.

Put the processed veggie mixture into a tea towel and wring out excess liquid – this will help keep the meatballs firm. Transfer to a mixing bowl. Add the rest of the ingredients and mix until well combined. Form the mixture into medium-sized balls.

Put the balls in the fridge and let freeze for 2 hours so that they can firm up.

Put the balls in the air fryer basket. Set the temperature to 160C and set the timer for 10 minutes. After 10 minutes, turn the balls. Set the temperature to 200C and the timer for 10 minutes.

Notes: If the meatball mixture is not sticking well enough to form into balls, add a little bit more oats to stiffen it – apply the oats accordingly.

211. Avocado Fries

Servings: 3

Preparation Time: 10 minutes

Cooking Time: 10 minutes

Ingredients:

1 Haas avocado, peeled, pitted, and sliced

1/2 cup panko breadcrumbs

1/2 teaspoon salt

Aquafaba from 1 can (15 ounces) garbanzo beans or white beans

Directions:

Put the salt and panko breadcrumbs into a shallow bowl and toss to mix.

Dredge the slices of avocado in the aquafaba and then coat with the panko mixture, covering them evenly well.

In a single layer, arrange the coated slices in the air fryer basket – DO NOT OVERLAP.

Set the temperature to 390F and the timer for 10 minutes. Shake well after 5 minutes.

Serve right away with your favorite vegan dipping sauce.

212. Oil-Free Vegan Samosa

Servings: 2-4

Preparation Time: 30 minutes

Cooking Time: 6 minutes

Ingredients:

For the potato filling:

1 clove garlic, crushed

1 onion, small-sized, finely chopped

1 potato, medium-sized, peeled and then mashed

1 teaspoon cumin powder

1 teaspoon ground coriander

1/2 cup carrots and pea mixture - frozen is okay

1/2-1 teaspoon curry powder

1/4 teaspoon turmeric powder

2 teaspoons organic coconut oil

Sea salt, to taste

Black pepper, to taste

For the cheese filling:

4 sheets rice paper

2 tablespoons Tofutti cream cheese

2 tablespoons parsley, finely chopped

1 teaspoon lemon juice

1 teaspoon extra virgin olive oil

1 tablespoon nutritional yeast

1 serving (3 ounces) firm tofu

Black pepper, to taste

Sea salt, to taste

Chili powder, to taste, optional

Directions:

Put the coconut oil in a medium-sized pot and heat. When the oil is hot, add the coriander, cumin, curry powder, and onion, and then sauté until translucent.

Add the carrots and peas, and then stir over medium heat for a couple of minutes.

Add the mashed potato and turmeric. Season with pepper and salt to taste, and then using a fork, mix well until combined. Set aside to cool.

Get a large-sized shallow tray and fill with lukewarm water. One piece at a time, soak the rice paper for a couple of seconds and then put on a clean cutting board. Using a sharp knife, cut the sheet into halves – slice the sheet before it gets completely soft, creating 2 half-circle pieces that are starting to soften.

Spoon 1 tablespoon or more of the filling mixture in the corner of 1 sheet. Fold the sheet in alternating directions, making a triangle and then roll the loose ends of the sheet to seal. Repeat the process with the remaining sheets and filling.

Put the samosa triangles into the air fryer basket and cook at 200C for 6 minutes.

Serve right away.

213. Vegan Bacon Wrapped Mini Breakfast Burritos

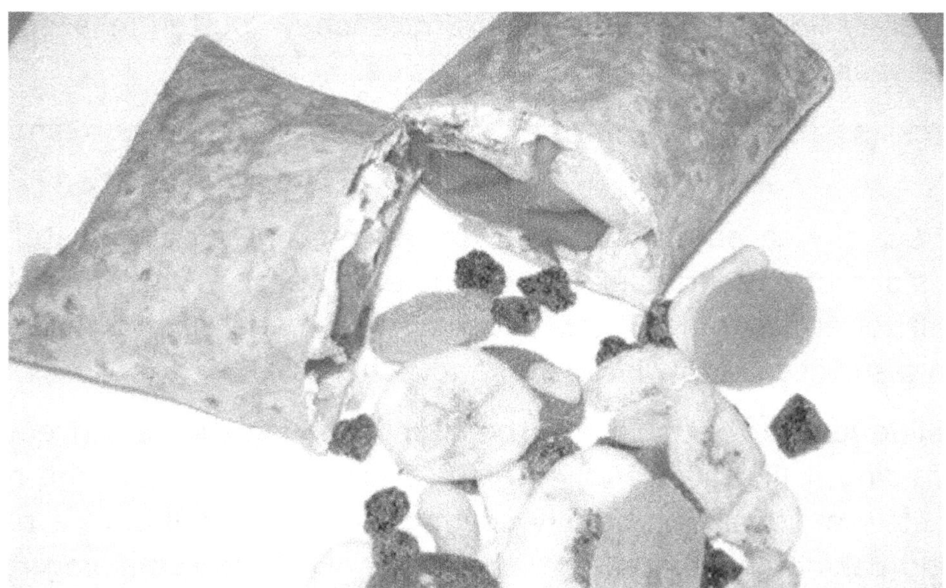

Servings: 4

Preparation Time: 20 minutes

Cooking Time: 8-10 minutes

Ingredients:

1-2 tablespoons liquid smoke

1-2 tablespoons water

2of your favorite tofu scramble or vegan egg scramble

2 tablespoons cashew butter

2-3 tablespoons tamari

4 pieces of rice paper

Vegetable add-ins:

8 strips of roasted red pepper

6-8 stalks fresh asparagus

1 small tree broccoli, sautéed

1/3 cup roasted sweet potato cubes

Handful kale, spinach, and/or other greens

Directions:

Put the water, liquid smoke, tamari, and cashew butter in a small-sized, shallow bowl and whisk to combine. Set aside.

Ready a clean surface or a large-sized plate for filling and rolling the rice paper.

Hold a sheet of rice paper under the faucet of cool running water, wetting both the sides of the wrapper for a couple of seconds until wet – the rice papers will soften more as it sits, but they will not get too soft that they will stick onto a surface or rip when you handle them.

Put the filling just in the middle of the sheet, leaving the sides free. Fold the 2 sides, folding it like a burrito, roll into a log, and seal. Dip the roll in the cashew butter mixture, completely coating it. Put the roll onto a parchment paper-lined baking sheet. Repeat the process with the remaining rolls filling and rice paper sheet. Set the temperature to 350F and the timer for 8 to 10 minutes, or till the rice papers are crisp.

214. Fried Sweet Potato And Homemade Guacamole

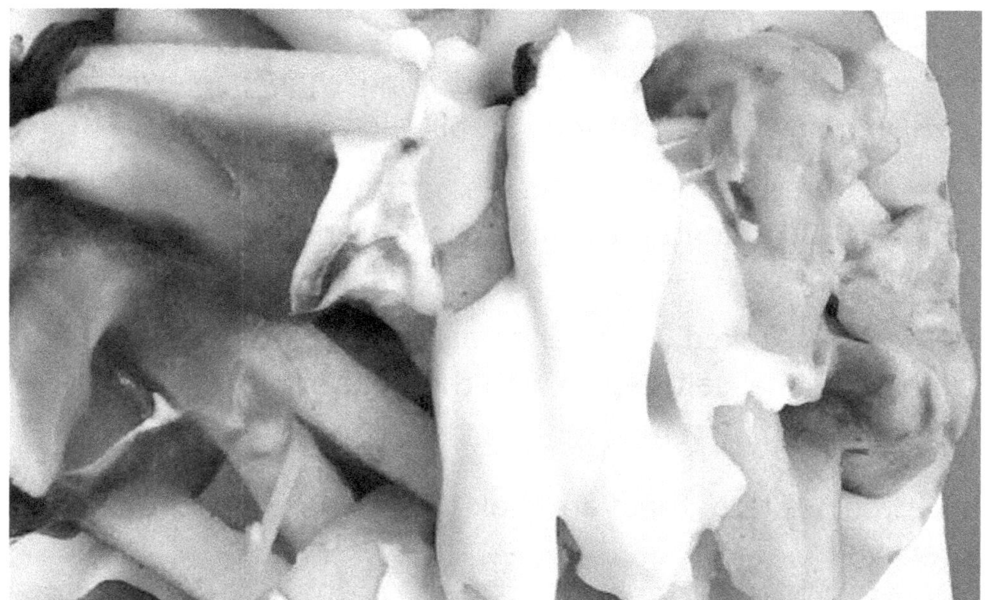

Servings: 2

Preparation Time: 15 minutes

Cooking Time: 30 minutes

Ingredients:

For the fries:

1-2 sweet potatoes, medium-sized, washed and peel left on

1 tablespoon of coconut oil, melted

For the guacamole:

1 bunch of fresh herbs, roughly chopped, I used rosemary, oregano, and parsley

1 ripe avocado, large-sized

1 sized cucumber, medium-sized, sliced and diced

1 sized tomato, medium-sized, sliced and diced

1 teaspoon garlic powder

Himalayan Pink Salt, to taste

Pepper, to taste

Directions:

For the fries:

Slice the sweet potatoes lengthwise into long-shaped pieces and then put them in a mixing bowl. Add the coconut oil and toss to coat.

Put into the air fryer basket. Set the temperature to 375F or 190C and set the timer for 20-30 minutes or until cooked and golden – shake halfway through cooking.

When the fries are cooked, transfer to a serving platter or serving bowl and sprinkle with additional salt. Serve with the guacamole.

For the guacamole:

While the sweet potato fries are baking, prepare all the ingredients as described above.

Slice the avocado into halves; discard the seeds and pith. Put the avocado meat in a mixing bowl and mash to desired consistency.

Add the rest of the ingredients and stir to combine. Refrigerate until the fries are cooked.

215. Corn Tortilla Chips

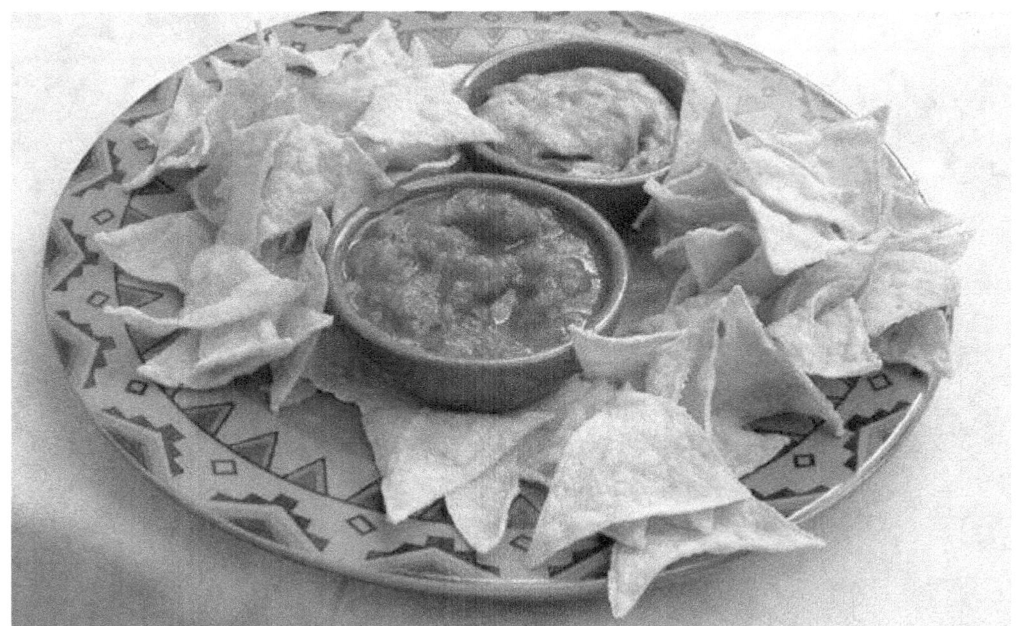

Servings: 2

Preparation Time: 1 minute

Cooking Time: 3 minutes

Ingredients:

8 corn tortillas

1 tablespoon of olive oil

Salt, to taste

Directions:

Preheat the air fryer to 200C.

Using a sharp knife, slice the corn tortillas into triangles. Brush all the triangles with the olive oil.

Put half the tortilla pieces in the air fryer basket and set the timer for 3 minutes.

Repeat the process with the remaining half.

Sprinkle the cooked tortilla with the salt. Serve with salsa, guacamole, or your preferred dip.

216. Crispy Vegetable Fries Fries

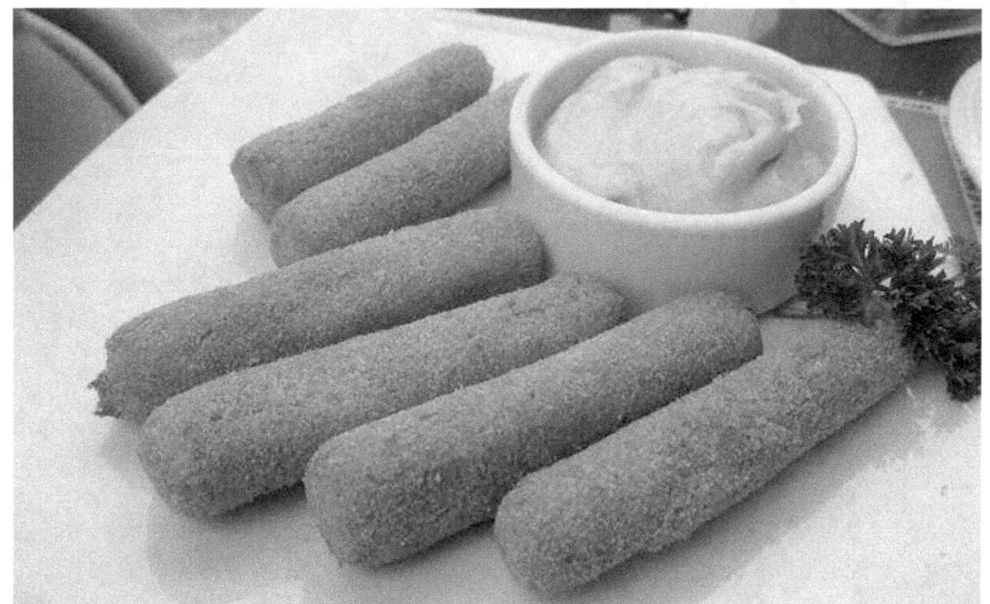

Servings: 4

Preparation Time: 15 minutes

Cooking Time: 8 minutes

Ingredients:

1 cup of panko breadcrumbs (regular or gluten-free)

1 cup rice flour

2 tablespoons Vegan Egg powder (I used Follow Your Heart)

2 tablespoons nutritional yeast flakes, divided

2/3 cup cold water

Assorted vegetables of your choice, sliced into shapes similar to French fry or into bite-size chunks (such as green beans, cauliflower, zucchini, sweet onions, or squash)

Salt and pepper

Directions:

Prepare 3 pieces of shallow dishes on a counter. Put rice flour in 1 of the dish. In the second dish, whisk the egg powder with 2/3 cup water and 1 tablespoon nutritional yeast until the mixture is smooth. In the third dish, mix the panko breadcrumbs with the remaining 1 tablespoon nutritional yeast and then add a couple pinches pepper and salt.

Working 1 vegetable piece at a time, coat with rice flour, into the vegan egg mixture, and finally in the breadcrumb mix, pressing to set the coating. Prepare as many veggies as you desire.

Lightly spritz the air fryer with oil. Alternatively, you can line the air fryer basket with parchment paper that is smaller than the basket. Carefully put the coated veggies in the air fryer basket and gently spritz with oil. Set the temperature to 380F and the timer for 8 minutes. Cook for additional minutes, if needed.

Serve while still crispy and hot with your choice of dipping sauce.

217. Buffalo Cauliflower

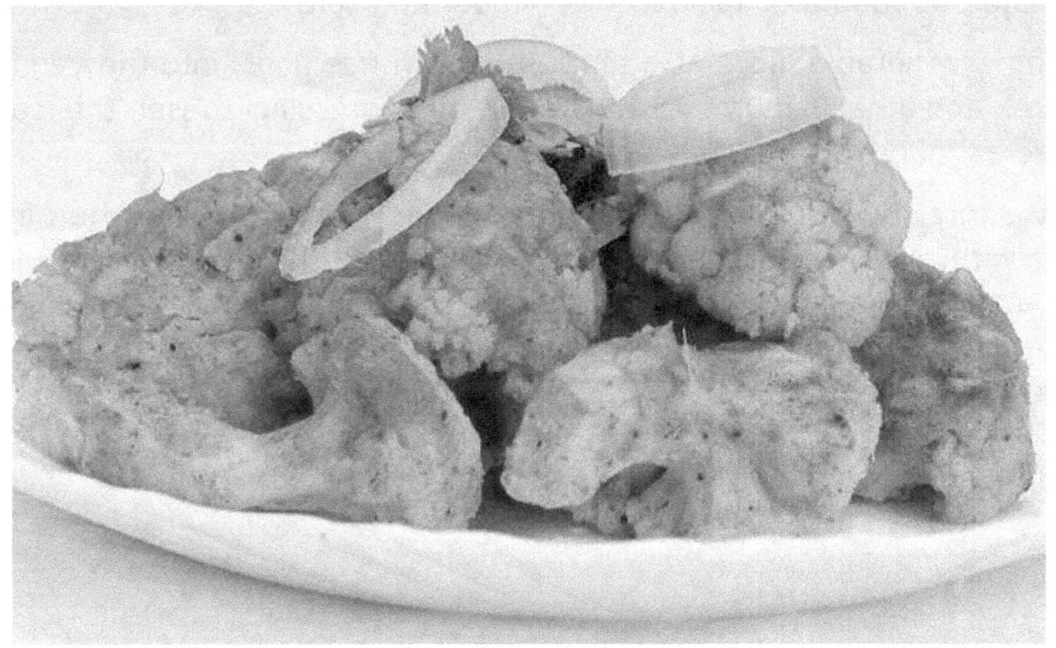

Servings: 4

Preparation Time: 5 minutes

Cooking Time: 15 minutes

Ingredients:

For the cauliflower:

4 cups cauliflower florets – use florets that are the size of 2 pieces baby carrots put side-by-side

1 cup panko breadcrumbs

1 teaspoon sea salt – DO NOT USE REGULAR SALT

For the Buffalo coating:

1/4 cup vegan Buffalo sauce (I used Frank's Red Hot) - Check the ingredients for butter

1/4 cup vegan butter, melted measurement

For dipping:

Vegan mayo Cashew Ranch, or your favorite creamy salad dressing

Directions:

Put the vegan butter in a microwavable mug and microwave to melt. Add the buffalo sauce and whisk to combine.

Combine the panko breadcrumbs with the salt in a shallow bowl.

Hold a floret by the stem, dip into the Buffalo coating, making sure that the floret is coated with the sauce – it's perfectly fine if the stem isn't coated with the sauce. Hold the floret over the mug until the sauce stops dripping from it – few drips are okay, but the raining sauce is not since it will make the panko bread clumpy and stop sticking on the cauliflower.

Dredge the sauce-coated floret in the breadcrumb mixture, coating it as much as you like, and then put into the air fryer basket. Repeat the process with the remaining florets – no need to arrange them in a single layer in the basket, just put them in.

Set the temperature to 350F and set the timer for 14-17 minutes, shaking the basket a couple of times and checking the progress during the process. The cauliflower is cooked when the florets are browned a little bit. Serve with your choice of dipping sauce.

Notes: These do not stay crunchy for long, so eat them right away. If there are leftovers, reheat them in the air fryer to make them crunchy again.

218. Garlic Rice Stuffed Mushrooms

Preparation Time: 5 minutes

Cooking Time: 15 minutes

Servings: 4

Ingredients:

1 cup cooked short grain rice

½ cup black beans, drained and rinsed

3 cloves garlic, minced

1 tsp coriander powder

Salt and freshly ground black pepper

1 tbsp olive oil + extra for drizzling

½ tbsp chopped parsley

½ tbsp. chopped oregano

16 small button mushrooms cups

Directions:

In a bowl, mix all the ingredients except the mushroom caps.

Preheat the air fryer.

In each mushroom cup, spoon the rice mixture to the brim of the mushrooms.

Drizzle with some olive oil and place 5 to 6 mushrooms in the fryer basket.

Slide the basket into the air fryer and bake at 370 F for 10 to 15 minutes or until the mushrooms nicely brown.

Transfer to a plate when ready and cook the remaining mushrooms.

Garnish with extra parsley and serve warm with tomato sauce.

Nutrition:

Calories 300

Total Fat 20g

Total Carbs 23g

Fiber 7g

Net Carbs 16g

Protein 8g

219. Winter Vegetable Roast

Preparation Time: 15 minutes

Cooking Time: 12 minutes

Servings: 4

Ingredients:

1 butternut squash, peeled and cubed

2 sweet potatoes, peeled and diced

2 potatoes, peeled and diced

3 large carrots, peeled and cut into chunks

1 tbsp fresh thyme leaves

1 tbsp fresh rosemary leaves

4 tbsp olive oil

Salt to taste

Directions:

In a bowl, combine all the ingredients and toss to coat.

Preheat the air fryer.

Pour half of the vegetables in the fryer basket and roast at 370 F for 10 to 12 minutes or until the vegetables are tender. Shake the basket halfway.

Spoon the vegetables into serving bowls and cook the remaining.

Serve warm with mustard drizzling sauce.

Nutrition:

Calories 131

Total Fat 3g

Total Carbs 26g

Fiber 11g

Net Carbs 15g

Protein 2g

220. Apple And Walnuts Mini Pizza

Preparation Time: 7 minutes

Cooking Time: 10 minutes

Servings: 4

Ingredients:

4 French flat bread (choose a size to fit into your fryer basket)

2 tbsp olive oil

1 tsp nutmeg powder

1 cup grated vegan mozzarella cheese

2 red apples, sliced thinly

1 cup crumbled vegan goat cheese

½ cup chopped walnuts

1 tsp dried thyme

Directions:

Lay the bread on a flat surface, brush with olive oil, and sprinkle with nutmeg powder.

Sprinkle with mozzarella cheese, share the apple slices on top, and sprinkle with the goat cheese, and walnuts.

One after the other, bake the pizza in the air fryer at 350 F for 10 minutes or until the mozzarella melts.

Remove onto a plate and cook the remaining pizza.

Slice into 4 wedges each, sprinkle with thyme and serve.

Nutrition:

Calories 139

Total Fat 2g

Total Carbs 27g

Fiber 3g

Net Carbs 24g

Protein 3g

221. Creamy Eggplant Gratin

Preparation Time: 10 minutes

Cooking Time: 25 minutes

Servings: 4

Ingredients:

¼ cup coconut cream

½ cup vegan parmesan cheese

½ cup marinara sauce

1 large eggplant, cut into ½ -inch slices

Salt and freshly ground black pepper to taste

Directions:

In a bowl, mix the coconut cream with the vegan parmesan cheese.

Then, grease a 3 x 3 baking dish with cooking spray and layer in half of the eggplant slices.

Spread half of the marinara sauce on top followed by the cream mixture. Season with salt and black pepper. Repeat the layers a second time to exhaust the ingredients.

Preheat the air fryer and carefully place the dish in the fryer basket.

Bake the gratin at 400 F for 20 to 25 minutes or until the cheese is golden brown on top.

Remove the dish; allow cooling for a few minutes.

Serve the gratin.

Nutrition facts per serving

Calories 344

Total Fat 20g

Total Carbs 28g

Fiber 0g

Net Carbs 28g

Protein 13g

222. Parmesan Heirloom Carrots Fries

Preparation Time: 5 minutes

Cooking Time: 8 minutes

Servings: 4

Ingredients:

8 heirloom carrots

1 tbsp olive oil

Salt and freshly ground black pepper

¼ cup grated vegan parmesan cheese

Chopped fresh parsley to garnish

Directions:

Cut the carrots in half widthwise and julienned lengthwise.

Combine all the ingredients in a bowl except the parsley and toss well.

Preheat the air fryer and pour half of the carrots into the fryer basket.

Fry at 350 F for 8 minutes, shaking the basket halfway.

Plate the carrots and garnish with the parsley.

Serve with your preferred dipping sauce.

Nutrition:

Calories 30

Total Fat 0.2g

Total Carbs 7g

Fiber 2g

Net Carbs 5g

Protein 1g

223. Stuffed Peppers With Quinoa And Black Beans

Preparation Time: 10 minutes

Cooking Time: 10 minutes

Servings: 4

Ingredients:

1 cup cooked quinoa

1 cup canned black beans, drained and rinsed

½ cup salsa

1 tsp garlic powder

1 tsp cumin powder

1 tsp chili powder

1 cup canned corn kernel, drained

Salt and freshly ground black pepper to taste

1 tbsp olive oil

4 large red bell peppers

Directions:

In a bowl, mix all the ingredients but the bell peppers. Set aside.

Stand the bell peppers and cut off a quarter of their heads. Remove the seeds and ribs.

After, spoon the quinoa mixture into the peppers.

Preheat the air fryer and place the peppers in the fryer basket.

Bake the peppers at 380 F for 10 minutes or until the peppers are slightly softened and the filling browns a bit.

Remove the hot peppers onto a plate; allow cooling for a few minutes.

Serve with some salsa and avocados.

Nutrition:

Calories 279

Total Fat 9g

Total Carbs 36g

Fiber 10g

Net Carbs 26g

Protein 14g

224. Ginger Cauliflower Steak

Preparation Time: 7 minutes

Cooking Time: 12 minutes

Servings: 4

Ingredients:

2 medium cauliflowers

1 tsp turmeric powder

1 tsp ginger puree

Salt and freshly ground black pepper

¼ tsp cumin powder

2 tbsp coconut oil

Directions:

Use a knife to cut off the green leaves on the cauliflowers. Stand the vegetable and cut from top to bottom and through the core into 4 steaks each. Set aside.

In a bowl, mix the spices with the coconut oil.

Brush the cauliflower steaks on both sides with the mixture making sure each corner is touched with spice.

Place 4 steaks in the fryer basket and grill at 390 F for 12 minutes; turn halfway.

Plate the steaks and grill the rest.

After, serve with chipotle sauce and arugula-tomato salad.

Nutrition:

Calories 72

Total Fat 4g

Total Carbs 8g

Fiber 3g

Net Carbs 5g

Protein 2g

225. Sweet Potato And Beans Burger

Preparation Time: 10 minutes

Cooking Time: 12 minutes

Servings: 4

Ingredients:

1 cup canned black beans, drained and rinsed

2 cups mashed sweet potatoes

1 cup cooked quinoa

Salt and black pepper to taste

½ cup almond meal

1 tsp smoked paprika

½ cup chopped green onion

To assemble:

4 buns, halved

4 lettuce leaves

4 slices tomatoes

Directions:

Mash half of the black beans in a medium bowl and combine with the remaining patties ingredients including the whole beans. Mold four cakes out of the mixture. If too soft, mix with 1 to 2 tablespoons more of almond meal.

Preheat the air fryer and place 2 patties in the fryer basket. Oil lightly with cooking spray and bake at 390 F for 12 minutes. Flip after 7 minutes.

Remove onto a plate and bake the remaining.

To assemble, line four bottom halves of each bun with lettuce leaves, place a patty on each and top with a slice of tomato each. Cover with the other bun halves and serve immediately.

Nutrition:

Calories 222

Total Fat 6g

Total Carbs 34g

Fiber 10g

Net Carbs 24g

Protein 9g

226. Sweet, Sticky Riblets

Preparation Time: 10 minutes

Cooking Time: 20 minutes

Servings: 4

Ingredients:

8 seitan slices

1 cup barbecue sauce

1 tbsp tamarind concentrate

½ tsp sesame oil

Directions:

Preheat the air fryer.

Score the seitan with a knife and wrap in foil.

Place in the fryer basket and grill at 350 F for 15 minutes.

While the seitan cooks, in a bowl, combine the barbecue sauce, tamarind concentrate, and sesame oil.

Carefully remove the seitan when ready and take off the foil. Brush each piece thoroughly with the barbecue sauce mixture.

Return the seitan pieces to the fryer basket and cook again at 350 F for 5 minutes.

Plate the riblets and serve warm.

Tip: Once the fryer basket cools, immediately soak in soapy water and scrub with a soft sponge. Also, wipe the air fryer clean with a wet napkin to prevent the barbecue sauce from drying in it.

Nutrition:

Calories 88

Total Fat 1g

Total Carbs 8g

Fiber 1g

Net Carbs 7g

Protein 11g

227. Coconut Crusted Fishless Fillets

Preparation Time: 10 minutes

Cooking Time: 10 minutes

Servings: 2

Ingredients:

2 flax seed powder + 6 tbsp water

2 tbsp olive oil

A pinch of salt

1 cup shredded coconut

4 fishless fillets

Directions:

In a bowl, mix the flaxseed powder with water and allow thickening for 5 minutes.

In another bowl, combine the olive oil, salt, and coconut.

Preheat the air fryer.

Dip the fishless fillets lightly in the flax egg and coat generously in the coconut mixture.

Place two fillets in the fryer basket and fry at 390 F for 10 minutes, flipping halfway.

Put the crusted fillets in a plate and cook the remaining.

Serve when ready with heirloom carrots fries.

Nutrition:

Calories 180

Total Fat 11g

Total Carbs 12g

Fiber 3g

Net Carbs 9g

Protein 9g

228. Broccoli Tofu Stir Fry

Preparation Time: 33 minutes

Cooking Time: 12 minutes

Servings: 4

Ingredients:

2 tbsp soy sauce

½ tsp sriracha hot sauce

1 tsp plain vinegar

1 tsp stevia sweetener

1 tbsp peanut butter

3 cloves garlic, minced

1 tbsp olive oil

1 lb extra firm tofu, pressed

2 cups broccoli florets

1 large red bell pepper, seeded and cut into strips

Directions:

In a bowl, mix all the ingredients except the tofu, broccoli florets, and bell peppers, and divide the sauce into two bowls.

Cut the tofu into cubes and toss with half of the sauce. Cover the bowl with plastic wrap and marinate in the fridge for 30 minutes.

Add the broccoli and bell pepper to the other sauce, mix, and allow sitting for a few minutes.

Preheat the air fryer after 30 minutes.

Remove the tofu from the fridge and use a slotted spoon to fetch the tofu into the fryer basket. (Drip as much liquid as possible from the tofu)

Cook at 360 F for 5 minutes, turning halfway. Use tongs to remove into a bowl after.

Fetch the broccoli into the fryer basket draining most of the liquid. Reduce the temperature to 200 F and cook for 7 minutes. Shake the basket after 5 minutes.

Combine the broccoli with the tofu, sprinkle with sesame seeds, and serve with white rice.

Nutrition:

Calories 151

Total Fat 7g

Total Carbs 13g

Fiber 3g

Net Carbs 10g

Protein 8g

229. Chickpea Cauliflower Tacos

Preparation Time: 5 minutes

Cooking Time: 20 minutes

Servings: 2

Ingredients:

1 tsp Mexican seasoning

1 (15 oz) can chickpea, drained and rinsed

2 cups cauliflower florets

Salt and freshly ground black pepper to taste

4 corn tortillas

1 cup shredded red cabbage

1 avocado, pitted and sliced

1 jalapeno, sliced and seeded

Dairy free sour cream for topping

Directions:

Mix the Mexican seasoning with the chickpeas, cauliflower, salt, and black pepper.

Preheat the air fryer and spoon the chickpeas and cauliflower into the fryer basket. Roast at 350 F for 20 minutes, shaking the basket halfway.

When ready, spoon the mixture into a bowl and assemble the tacos.

Share the chickpeas and cauliflower into the corn tortillas. Top with the cabbage, jalapeno, and avocado.

Drizzle the sour cream on top and serve immediately.

Nutrition:

Calories 190

Total Fat 15g

Total Carbs 11g

Fiber 0g

Net Carbs 11g

Protein 3g

230. Patatas Bravas

Preparation Time: 15 minutes

Cooking Time: 28 minutes

Servings: 4

Ingredients:

4 large potatoes, peeled and chopped

Salt and black pepper to taste

1 small red onion, chopped

3 tsp Italian mixed herbs

1 tomato thinly sliced

1 tsp sweet paprika

1 tsp chili powder

2 tbsp olive oil

1 cup tomato sauce

1 tbsp red wine vinegar

Directions:

Pour the potatoes in the fryer basket, oil with cooking spray, and cook at 350 F for 20 minutes or until the vegetables are tender.

Fetch into a bowl and set aside.

Mix the remaining ingredients in a 3 x 3 baking dish and put into the fryer basket. Cook at 350 F for 8 minutes.

When ready, pour the sauce over the potatoes and serve.

Nutrition:

Calories 126

Total Fat 4g

Total Carbs 20g

Fiber 2g

Net Carbs 18g

Protein 2g

231. Couscous Stuffed Eggplants

Preparation Time: 4 minutes

Cooking Time: 10 minutes

Servings: 2

Ingredients:

1 eggplant, halved

1 cup cooked couscous

1 tbsp olive oil

1 garlic powder

1 onion powder

1 tomato, chopped

2 tbsp chopped parsley

2 tbsp black currants

Salt and freshly ground black pepper

½ cup vegan feta cheese, crumbled

Directions:

Scoop the pulp of the eggplants and chop. Put in a bowl and mix with the remaining ingredients except for the feta cheese.

Spoon the filling into the eggplant halves and scatter the feta cheese on top.

Preheat the air fryer and place the eggplants in the fryer basket.

Bake at 350 F for 10 minutes or until the eggplant is tender.

When ready, remove and serve with baby green salad.

Nutrition:

Calories 320

Total Fat 6g

Total Carbs 56g

Fiber 13g

Net Carbs 43g

Protein 11g

232. Bean Quinoa Zucchini Boats

Preparation Time: 4 minutes

Cooking Time: 10 minutes

Servings: 4

Ingredients:

2 zucchinis, halved

1 cup canned black beans, drained and rinsed

1 cup cooked quinoa

Salt and freshly ground black pepper to taste

1 garlic clove, minced

1 tbsp olive oil

Directions:

Scoop the pulp of the zucchinis and chop. Put in a bowl.

Add the remaining ingredients, mix, and spoon the mixture into the zucchini boats.

Preheat the air fryer and place two zucchinis in the fryer basket.

Bake at 350 F for 10 minutes or until the zucchinis are tender.

Plate after and cook the other two.

Serve warm with tomato avocado salad.

Nutrition:

Calories 193

Total Fat 5g

Total Carbs 32g

Fiber 4g

Net Carbs 29g

Protein 5g

233. Tofu Nuggets

Preparation Time: 8 minutes

Cooking Time: 15 minutes

Servings: 4

Ingredients:

6 tbsp soymilk

1 tsp salt

1 tsp garlic powder

3 tbsp Dijon mustard

4 tbsp flour

2 tsp Italian seasoning blend

1 cup breadcrumbs

1/3 cup cornmeal

14 oz extra firm tofu, pressed

Directions:

In a bowl, mix the soymilk, garlic powder, Dijon mustard, flour, and seasoning blend. Set aside.

Also, combine the breadcrumbs and cornmeal in a different bowl.

Cut the tofu into slices.

Preheat the air fryer. When ready, dip some tofu slices into the milk batter and coat in the cornmeal mixture. Place in the fryer basket without overlapping.

Air fry the tofu at 400 F for 15 minutes, turning halfway.

Transfer to a plate; coat and cook the remaining tofu.

Divide into four dishes and serve warm with sweet chili sauce, and cabbage salad.

Nutrition:

Calories 80

Total Fat 3g

Total Carbs 11g

Fiber 0g

Net Carbs 11g

Protein 3g

234. Three Veg Bake

Preparation Time: 15 minutes

Cooking Time: 15 minutes

Servings: 2

Ingredients:

3 red bell peppers, seeded and cut into chunks

1 large red onion, cut into wedges

1 large zucchini, cut into wedges

1 tbsp olive oil

Salt and freshly ground black pepper

2 cloves garlic, crushed

1 bay leaf, cut into 6 pieces

Directions:

Put the bell pepper, onion, and zucchini in a bowl. Drizzle with olive oil and season with salt and black pepper.

Preheat the air fryer.

In a 3 x 3 baking dish, pour in the vegetables, slip the bay leaves into different parts of the bowl, and tuck in the garlic likewise.

Place the dish in the fryer basket and cook at 330 F for 15 minutes.

Once ready, remove, and discard the bay leaves and garlic.

Serve the dish warm.

Nutrition:

Calories 95

Total Fat 8g

Total Carbs 4g

Fiber 2g

Net Carbs 2g

Protein 2g

235. Roasted Balsamic Brussel Sprouts

Preparation Time: 10 minutes

Cooking Time: 30 minutes

Servings: 4

Ingredients:

1 lb Brussels sprouts, trimmed and halved

Hot water for blanching

Salt and freshly black pepper to taste

1 ½ tbsp melted vegan butter

1 tsp garlic powder

1 tbsp balsamic vinegar

Directions:

In a bowl, add the Brussels sprouts to the hot water and blanch for 3 minutes, then, drain through a colander.

Preheat the air fryer.

In the strainer, toss the Brussels sprouts with salt, black pepper, vegan butter, garlic powder, and balsamic vinegar.

Pour the vegetables into the fryer basket and roast at 360 F for 10 minutes.

When ready, dish and serve warm with grilled tempeh.

Nutrition:

Calories 95

Total Fat 7g

Total Carbs 4g

Fiber 1g

Net Carbs 3g

Protein 3g

236. Roasted Heirloom Tomatoes

Preparation Time: 15 minutes

Cooking Time: 10 minutes

Servings: 2

Ingredients:

1 clove garlic

1 ½ tbsp. toasted pecans

¼ cup chopped cilantro

¼ cup chopped basil

Salt to taste

2 tsp + ¼ cup olive oil

2 heirloom tomato, halved

1 small white onion, thinly sliced

¼ cup grated vegan parmesan cheese

Directions:

In a food processor, add the garlic, pecans, cilantro, basil, and salt. Process at slow speed while adding the quarter cup of olive oil slowly. Pour the pesto into a bowl.

Pat the tomato dry with paper towel and spread half of the pesto on top.

Toss the onion with the remaining olive oil and spoon onto the tomato. Then, sprinkle with the vegan parmesan cheese.

Carefully place two tomatoes in the fryer basket and grill at 300 F for 10 minutes.

Remove the tomato onto a serving plate and cook the other two tomatoes.

When ready, season all four tomatoes with salt, and spread the remaining pesto on top.

Serve it with steamed green beans.

Nutrition:

Calories 168

Total Fat 15g

Total Carbs 5g

Fiber 2g

Net Carbs 3g

Protein 4g

237. Baked Cajun Tempeh

Preparation Time: 2 minutes

Cooking Time: 8 minutes

Servings: 4

Ingredients:

8 tempeh slices

1 tbsp olive oil

1 tsp Cajun seasoning

½ tsp cayenne pepper

Directions:

Preheat the air fryer.

Brush the tempeh on both sides with olive oil and season with Cajun and cayenne pepper.

Place 4 tempeh slices in the fryer basket, and bake at 390 F for 8 minutes.

Remove onto a plate and cook the remaining tempeh.

Serve with tomato - avocado salad.

Nutrition:

Calories 319

Total Fat 21g

Total Carbs 20g

Fiber 3g

Net Carbs 17g

Protein 13g

238. Mixed Vegetable Bowls

Preparation Time: 30 minutes

Cooking Time: 1 hour 10 minutes

Servings: 4

Ingredients:

1 cup cauliflower florets

1 cup broccoli florets

1 small zucchini, chopped

2 tbsp garlic-ginger puree

1 tbsp onion powder

2 tbsp olive oil

1 tbsp curry paste

2 tsp mixed spice

1 ½ cups coconut milk

Salt and freshly ground black pepper as needed

Directions:

In a medium bowl, combine the cauliflower, broccoli, zucchini, ginger-garlic paste, onion powder, olive oil, curry paste, mixed spices, and coconut milk. Stir to be well mixed.

Cover the bowl with a plastic wrap and refrigerate for 1 hour to marinate the vegetables.

Preheat the air fryer.

Remove the veggies from the fridge and use a slotted spoon to fetch some vegetables into the fryer basket making sure to drip off as much liquid as possible.

Crisp the veggies at 350 F for 10 minutes or until softened and golden brown.

Spoon the vegetables into a serving bowl and serve with coconut sauce.

Nutrition:

Calories 160

Total Fat 15g

Total Carbs 3g

Fiber 1g

Net Carbs 2g

Protein 3g

239. Thyme Roast Vegetables

Preparation Time: 15 minutes

Cooking Time: 16 minutes

Servings: 4

Ingredients:

1 small parsnip, peeled and sliced into 2-inch cubes

2 small red onions, cut into wedges

1 cup chopped butternut squash

1 tbsp chopped fresh thyme

Salt and freshly ground black pepper to taste

2 tsp melted vegan butter

Directions:

Preheat the air fryer.

In a bowl, mix the parsnips, onions, butternut squash, thyme, salt, black pepper, and vegan butter.

Pour the vegetables into the fryer basket and cook at 200 F for 16 minutes.

Transfer the roasted veggies into a serving bowl, season with salt as desired, and serve immediately.

Nutrition:

Calories 50

Total Fat 3g

Sodium 30mg

Total Carbs 5g

Net Carbs 3g

Protein 2g

240. Eggplant Bake

Preparation Time: 10 minutes

Cooking Time: 20 minutes

Servings: 4

Ingredients:

1 cup cubed eggplant

1/3 cup chopped tomatoes

¼ cup chopped red bell pepper

¼ cup chopped green bell pepper

¼ cup chopped yellow onion

1 clove garlic, minced

1 tbsp sliced pimento olives

¼ tsp dried basil

¼ tsp dried marjoram

Salt and freshly ground black pepper to taste

¼ cup grated vegan mozzarella cheese

1 tbsp coconut flour breadcrumbs

Directions:

Preheat the air fryer.

In a bowl, mix the eggplant, tomatoes, bell peppers, onion, garlic, olives, basil, marjoram, salt, and black pepper.

Lightly grease a 3 x 3 baking dish with cooking spray and pour in the eggplant mixture. Level the top with a spatula.

Sprinkle with the vegan mozzarella cheese on top of it and followed by the breadcrumbs.

Place the dish in the fryer basket and cook at 300 F for 20 minutes.

When ready, remove and serve immediately.

Nutrition:

Calories 317

Total Fat 26g

Total Carbs 8g

Finer 4g

Net Carbs 6g

Protein 12g

241. Spinach Zucchini Frittata

Preparation Time: 15 minutes

Cooking Time: 15 minutes

Servings: 2

Ingredients:

4 eggs, cracked into a bowl

1/3 cup almond milk

Salt and freshly ground black pepper to taste

2 tsp vegan butter

1 cup baby spinach

1/3 cup sliced cremini mushrooms

1 small red onion, sliced

1 large zucchini, cut into 1-inch slices

¼ cup chopped green onions

¼ lb asparagus, trimmed and sliced thinly

1/3 cup grated vegan cheddar cheese

Directions:

Line a 3 x 3 baking dish with parchment paper and set aside.

Whisk the eggs with the almond milk, salt, and black pepper. Set aside.

Melt the vegan butter in a skillet over medium heat and sauté the spinach, mushrooms, onion, zucchini, green onions, and asparagus until softened about 8 minutes.

Pour the veggies into the baking dish and pour the egg mixture all over.

Sprinkle with the vegan cheddar cheese and place the bowl in the fryer basket. Cook at 320 F for 15 minutes.

When ready, remove the frittata, cut out slices, and serve.

Nutrition:

Calories 220

Total Fat 18g

Total Carbs 9g

Fiber 4g

Net Carbs 5g

Protein 6g

242. Fried Tofu Recipe From Malaysia

Servings: 4

Cooking Time: 30 minutes

Ingredients

1 block tofu, cut into strips

1 tablespoon maple syrup

1 teaspoon sriracha sauce

2 cloves of garlic

2 tablespoons soy sauce

2 teaspoons fresh ginger no need to peel, coarsely chopped

juice of 1 fresh lime

Peanut Butter Sauce Ingredients

1 tablespoon soy sauce

1/2 cup creamy peanut butter

1-2 teaspoons Sriracha sauce to taste

2 cloves of garlic

2-inch piece of fresh ginger coarsely chopped

6 tablespoons of water

juice of 1/2 a fresh lemon

Direction:

In a blender, blend all peanut butter sauce Ingredients: until smooth and creamy. Transfer to a medium bowl and set aside for dipping sauce.

In same blender, blend garlic, sriracha, ginger, maple syrup, lime juice, and soy sauce until smooth. Pour into a bowl and add strips of tofu, Marinate for 30 minutes.

With the steel skewer, skewer tofu strips.

Place on skewer rack and air fry for 15 minutes at 370oF.

Serve and enjoy.

Nutrition:

Calories: 347; Carbs: 16.6g; Protein: 16.6g; Fat: 23.8g

243. Pita 'N Tomato Pesto Casserole

Servings: 3

Cooking Time: 5 minutes

Ingredients

1 roma (plum) tomatoes, chopped

1 tablespoon and 1-1/2 teaspoons olive oil

1 tablespoon grated Parmesan cheese

1/2 bunch spinach, rinsed and chopped

1/4 cup crumbled feta cheese

2 fresh mushrooms, sliced

3 (6 inch) whole wheat pita breads

3-ounce sun-dried tomato pesto

ground black pepper to taste

Direction:

Lightly grease baking pan of air fryer with cooking spray.

Evenly spread tomato pesto on one side of pita bread. Place one pita bread on bottom of pan, add 1/3 each of Parmesan, feta, mushrooms, spinach, and tomatoes. Season with pepper and drizzle with olive oil.

Cook for 5 minutes at 390oF until tops crisped.

Repeat process for remaining pita bread.

Serve and enjoy.

Nutrition:

Calories: 367; Carbs: 41.6g; Protein: 11.6g; Fat: 17.1g

244. Baked Portobello, Pasta 'N Cheese

Servings: 4

Cooking Time: 30 minutes

Ingredients

1 cup milk

1 cup shredded mozzarella cheese

1 large clove garlic, minced

1 tablespoon vegetable oil

1/4 cup margarine

1/4 teaspoon dried basil

1/4-pound portobello mushrooms, thinly sliced

2 tablespoons all-purpose flour

2 tablespoons soy sauce

4-ounce penne pasta, cooked according to manufacturer's Directions for Cooking

5-ounce frozen chopped spinach, thawed

Direction:

Lightly grease baking pan of air fryer with oil. For 2 minutes, heat on 360oF. Add mushrooms and cook for a minute. Transfer to a plate.

In same pan, melt margarine for a minute. Stir in basil, garlic, and flour. Cook for 3 minutes. Stir and cook for another 2 minutes. Stir in half of milk slowly while whisking continuously. Cook for another 2 minutes. Mix well. Cook for another 2 minutes. Stir in remaining milk and cook for another 3 minutes.

Add cheese and mix well.

Stir in soy sauce, spinach, mushrooms, and pasta. Mix well. Top with remaining cheese.

Cook for 15 minutes at 390oF until tops are lightly browned.

Serve and enjoy.

Nutrition:

Calories: 482; Carbs: 32.1g; Protein: 16.0g; Fat: 32.1g

245. Layered Tortilla Bake

Servings: 6

Cooking Time: 30 minutes

Ingredients

1 (15 ounce) can black beans, rinsed and drained

1 cup salsa

1 cup salsa, divided

1/2 cup chopped tomatoes

1/2 cup sour cream

2 (15 ounce) cans pinto beans, drained and rinsed

2 cloves garlic, minced

2 cups shredded reduced-fat Cheddar cheese

2 tablespoons chopped fresh cilantro

7 (8 inch) flour tortillas

Direction:

Mash pinto beans in a large bowl and mix in garlic and salsa.

In another bowl whisk together tomatoes, black beans, cilantro, and ¼ cup salsa.

Lightly grease baking pan of air fryer with cooking spray. Spread 1 tortilla, spread ¾ cup pinto bean mixture evenly up to ½-inch away from the edge of tortilla, spread ¼ cup cheese on top. Cover with another tortilla, spread 2/3 cup black bean mixture, and then ¼ cup cheese. Repeat twice the layering process. Cover with the last tortilla, top with pinto bean mixture and then cheese.

Cover pan with foil.

Cook for 25 minutes at 390oF, remove foil and cook for 5 minutes or until tops are lightly browned.

Serve and enjoy.

Nutrition:

Calories: 409; Carbs: 54.8g; Protein: 21.1g; Fat: 11.7g

246. Baked Cheesy Eggplant With Marinara

Servings: 3

Cooking Time: 45 minutes

Ingredients

1 clove garlic, sliced

1 large eggplants

1 tablespoon olive oil

1 tablespoon olive oil

1/2 pinch salt, or as needed

1/4 cup and 2 tablespoons dry bread crumbs

1/4 cup and 2 tablespoons ricotta cheese

1/4 cup grated Parmesan cheese

1/4 cup grated Parmesan cheese

1/4 cup water, plus more as needed

1/4 teaspoon red pepper flakes

1-1/2 cups prepared marinara sauce

1-1/2 teaspoons olive oil

2 tablespoons shredded pepper jack cheese

salt and freshly ground black pepper to taste

Direction:

Cut eggplant crosswise in 5 pieces. Peel and chop two pieces into ½-inch cubes.

Lightly grease baking pan of air fryer with 1 tbsp olive oil. For 5 minutes, heat oil at 390oF. Add half eggplant strips and cook for 2 minutes per side. Transfer to a plate.

Add 1 ½ tsp olive oil and add garlic. Cook for a minute. Add chopped eggplants. Season with pepper flakes and salt. Cook for 4 minutes. Lower heat to 330oF and continue cooking eggplants until soft, around 8 minutes more.

Stir in water and marinara sauce. Cook for 7 minutes until heated through. Stirring every now and then. Transfer to a bowl.

In a bowl, whisk well pepper, salt, pepper jack cheese, Parmesan cheese, and ricotta. Evenly spread cheeses over eggplant strips and then fold in half.

Lay folded eggplant in baking pan. Pour marinara sauce on top.

In a small bowl whisk well olive oil, and bread crumbs. Sprinkle all over sauce.

Cook for 15 minutes at 390oF until tops are lightly browned.

Serve and enjoy.

Nutrition:

Calories: 405; Carbs: 41.1g; Protein: 12.7g; Fat: 21.4g

247. Baked Zucchini Recipe From Mexico

Servings: 4

Cooking Time: 30 minutes

Ingredients

1 tablespoon olive oil

1-1/2 pounds zucchini, cubed

1/2 cup chopped onion

1/2 teaspoon garlic salt

1/2 teaspoon paprika

1/2 teaspoon dried oregano

1/2 teaspoon cayenne pepper, or to taste

1/2 cup cooked long-grain rice

1/2 cup cooked pinto beans

1-1/4 cups salsa

3/4 cup shredded Cheddar cheese

Direction:

Lightly grease baking pan of air fryer with olive oil. Add onions and zucchini and for 10 minutes, cook on 360oF. Halfway through cooking time, stir.

Season with cayenne, oregano, paprika, and garlic salt. Mix well.

Stir in salsa, beans, and rice. Cook for 5 minutes.

Stir in cheddar cheese and mix well.

Cover pan with foil.

Cook for 15 minutes at 390oF until bubbly.

Serve and enjoy.

Nutrition:

Calories: 263; Carbs: 24.6g; Protein: 12.5g; Fat: 12.7g

248. Crisped Baked Cheese Stuffed Chile Pepper

Servings: 3

Cooking Time: 30 minutes

Ingredients

1 (7 ounce) can whole green Chile peppers, drained

1 egg, beaten

1 tablespoon all-purpose flour

1/2 (5 ounce) can evaporated milk

1/2 (8 ounce) can tomato sauce

1/4-pound Monterey Jack cheese, shredded

1/4-pound Longhorn or Cheddar cheese, shredded

1/4 cup milk

Direction:

Lightly grease baking pan of air fryer with cooking spray. Evenly spread chilies and sprinkle cheddar and Jack cheese on top.

In a bowl whisk well flour, milk, and eggs. Pour over chilies.

For 20 minutes, cook on 360oF.

Add tomato sauce on top.

Cook for 10 minutes at 390oF until tops are lightly browned.

Serve and enjoy.

Nutrition:

Calories: 392; Carbs: 12.0g; Protein: 23.9g; Fat: 27.6g

249. Creamy 'N Cheese Broccoli Bake

Servings: 2

Cooking Time: 30 minutes

Ingredients

1-pound fresh broccoli, coarsely chopped

2 tablespoons all-purpose flour

salt to taste

1 tablespoon dry bread crumbs, or to taste

1/2 large onion, coarsely chopped

1/2 (14 ounce) can evaporated milk, divided

1/2 cup cubed sharp Cheddar cheese

1-1/2 teaspoons butter, or to taste

1/4 cup water

Direction:

Lightly grease baking pan of air fryer with cooking spray. Mix in half of the milk and flour in pan and for 5 minutes, cook on 360oF. Halfway through cooking time, mix well. Add broccoli and remaining milk. Mix well and cook for another 5 minutes.

Stir in cheese and mix well until melted.

In a small bowl mix well, butter and bread crumbs. Sprinkle on top of broccoli.

Cook for 20 minutes at 360oF until tops are lightly browned.

Serve and enjoy.

Nutrition:

Calories: 444; Carbs: 37.3g; Protein: 23.1g; Fat: 22.4g

250. Buttered Carrot-Zucchini With Mayo

Servings: 4

Cooking Time: 25 minutes

Ingredients

1 tablespoon grated onion

2 tablespoons butter, melted

1/2-pound carrots, sliced

1-1/2 zucchinis, sliced

1/4 cup water

1/4 cup mayonnaise

1/4 teaspoon prepared horseradish

1/4 teaspoon salt

1/4 teaspoon ground black pepper

1/4 cup Italian bread crumbs

Direction:

Lightly grease baking pan of air fryer with cooking spray. Add carrots. For 8 minutes, cook on 360oF. Add zucchini and continue cooking for another 5 minutes.

Meanwhile, in a bowl whisk well pepper, salt, horseradish, onion, mayonnaise, and water. Pour into pan of veggies. Toss well to coat.

In a small bowl mix melted butter and bread crumbs. Sprinkle over veggies.

Cook for 10 minutes at 390oF until tops are lightly browned.

Serve and enjoy.

Nutrition:

Calories: 223; Carbs: 13.8g; Protein: 2.7g; Fat: 17.4g

251. Cheddar, Squash 'N Zucchini Casserole

Servings: 4

Cooking Time: 30 minutes

Ingredients

1 egg

5 saltine crackers, or as needed, crushed

2 tablespoons bread crumbs

1/2-pound yellow squash, sliced

1/2-pound zucchini, sliced

1/2 cup shredded Cheddar cheese

1-1/2 teaspoons white sugar

1/2 teaspoon salt

1/4 onion, diced

1/4 cup biscuit baking mix

1/4 cup butter

Direction:

Lightly grease baking pan of air fryer with cooking spray. Add onion, zucchini, and yellow squash. Cover pan with foil and for 15 minutes, cook on 360oF or until tender.

Stir in salt, sugar, egg, butter, baking mix, and cheddar cheese. Mix well. Fold in crushed crackers. Top with bread crumbs.

Cook for 15 minutes at 390oF until tops are lightly browned.

Serve and enjoy.

Nutrition:

Calories: 285; Carbs: 16.4g; Protein: 8.6g; Fat: 20.5g

252. Your Traditional Mac 'N Cheese

Servings: 3

Cooking Time: 32 minutes

Ingredients

1/2 pinch ground nutmeg

1/2 teaspoon Dijon mustard

1/2 teaspoon salt

1/4 cup panko bread crumbs

1/8 teaspoon cayenne pepper

1/8 teaspoon dried thyme

1/8 teaspoon white pepper

1/8 teaspoon Worcestershire sauce

1-1/2 cups milk

1-1/2 cups shredded sharp Cheddar cheese, divided

1-1/2 teaspoons butter, melted

2 tablespoons all-purpose flour

2 tablespoons butter

8-ounce elbow macaroni, cooked according to package Instructions

Direction:

Melt 2 tbsp butter in baking pan of air fryer for 2 minutes at 360oF. Stir in flour and cook for 3 minutes, stirring every now and then. Stir in white pepper, cayenne pepper, and thyme. Cook for 2 minutes. Stir in a cup of milk and whisk well. Cook for 5 minutes while mixing constantly.

Mix in salt, Worcestershire sauce, and nutmeg . Mix well. Cook for 5 minutes or until thickened while stirring frequently.

Add cheese and mix well. Cook for 3 minutes or until melted and thoroughly mixed.

Stir in Dijon mustard and mix well. Add macaroni and toss well to coat. Sprinkle remaining cheese on top.

In a small bowl mix well 1 ½ tsp butter and panko. Sprinkle on top of cheese.

Cook for 15 minutes at 390oF until tops are lightly browned.

Serve and enjoy.

Nutrition:

Calories: 700; Carbs: 72.8g; Protein: 29.4g; Fat: 32.3g

253. Shepherd's Pie Vegetarian Approved

Servings: 3

Cooking Time: 35 minutes

Top Layer Ingredients

2 tablespoons olive oil

1 teaspoon salt

2-1/2 russet potatoes, peeled and cut into 1-inch cubes

1 tablespoon and 1-1/2 teaspoons vegan cream cheese substitute (such as Tofutti ®)

1/4 cup vegan mayonnaise

1/4 cup soy milk

Bottom Layer Ingredients

1 carrot, chopped

1-1/2 teaspoons vegetable oil

1/2 large yellow onion, chopped

1-1/2 stalks celery, chopped

1/2 tomato, chopped

1/2 teaspoon Italian seasoning

1/2 clove garlic, minced, or more to taste

1/2 pinch ground black pepper to taste

1/2 (14 ounce) package vegetarian ground beef substitute

1/4 cup frozen peas

1/4 cup shredded Cheddar-style soy cheese

Direction:

Boil potatoes until tender. Drain and transfer to a bowl. Mash potatoes with salt, vegan cream cheese, olive oil, soy milk, and vegan mayonnaise. Mix well until smooth. Set aside.

Lightly grease baking pan of air fryer with cooking spray. Add carrot, celery, onions, tomato, and peas. For 10 minutes, cook on 360oF. Stirring halfway through cooking time.

Stir in pepper, garlic, and Italian seasoning.

Stir in vegetarian ground beef substitute. Cook for 5 minutes while halfway through cooking time crumbling and mixing the beef substitute.

Evenly spread the beef and veggie mixture in pan. Top evenly with mashed potato mixture.

Cook for another 20 minutes or until mashed potatoes are lightly browned.

Serve and enjoy.

Nutrition:

Calories: 559; Carbs: 64.5g; Protein: 20.2g; Fat: 24.4g

254. Loaded Brekky Hash Browns

Servings: 4

Cooking Time: 20 minutes

Ingredients

3 russet potatoes, peeled and grated

2 garlic cloves chopped

1 teaspoon paprika

salt and pepper to taste

1 teaspoon canola oil

1 teaspoon olive oil

1/4 cup chopped green peppers

1/4 cup chopped red peppers

1/4 cup chopped onions

Direction:

For 20 minutes, soak the grated potatoes in a bowl of cold water to make it crunchy and remove the starch. Then drain well and completely dry with paper towels.

Lightly grease baking pan of air fryer with cooking spray.

Add grated potatoes in air fryer. Season with garlic, paprika, salt, and pepper. Add canola and olive oil. Toss well to coat.

For 10 minutes, cook on 390oF.

Remove basket and toss the mixture a bit. Stir in green and red peppers, and onions.

Cook for another 10 minutes.

Serve and enjoy.

Nutrition:

Calories: 263; Carbs: 53.2g; Protein: 6.5g; Fat: 2.6g

255. Healthy Breakfast Casserole

Servings: 2

Cooking Time: 30 minutes

Ingredients

½ cup cooked quinoa

½ cup diced bell pepper

½ cup shiitake mushrooms, diced

½ tsp black pepper

½ tsp dill

½ tsp ground cumin

½ tsp red pepper flakes

½ tsp salt

1 large carrot, peeled and chopped

1 small onion, diced

1 tbsp lemon juice

1 tsp dried oregano

1 tsp garlic, minced

1 tsp olive oil

2 small celery stalks, chopped

2 tbsp soy yogurt, plain

2 tbsp water

2 tbsp yeast

7-oz extra firm tofu, drained

Direction:

Lightly grease baking pan of air fryer with olive oil. Add garlic and onion.

For 2 minutes, cook on 390oF.

Remove basket, stir in bell pepper, celery, and carrots. Cook for 3 minutes.

Remove basket, give a quick stir. Then add cumin, red pepper flakes, dill, pepper, salt, oregano, and mushrooms. Mix well. Cook for 5 minutes. Mixing halfway through cooking time.

Meanwhile, in a food processor pulse lemon juice, water, yogurt, yeast, and tofu. Process until creamy.

Transfer creamy tofu mixture into air fryer basket. Add quinoa and give a good stir.

Cook for another 15 minutes at 330oF or until golden brown.

Let it rest for 5 minutes.

Serve and enjoy.

Nutrition:

Calories: 280; Carbs: 28.6g; Protein: 18.5g; Fat: 10.1g

256. Skewered Corn In Air Fryer

Servings: 2

Cooking Time: 25 minutes

Ingredients

1-pound apricot, halved

2 ears of corn

2 medium green peppers, cut into large chunks

2 teaspoons prepared mustard

Salt and pepper to taste

Direction:

Preheat the air fryer to 3300F.

Place the grill pan accessory in the air fryer.

On the double layer rack with the skewer accessories, skewer the corn, green peppers, and apricot. Season with salt and pepper to taste.

Place skewered corn on the double layer rack and cook for 25 minutes.

Once cooked, brush with prepared mustard.

Nutrition:

Calories: 341; Carbs: 82.5g; Protein: 7.43g; Fat: 2.2g

257. Salted 'N Herbed Potato Packets

Servings: 3

Cooking Time: 40 minutes

Ingredients

1 ½ teaspoons seasoning blend

1 onion, sliced

2 large russet potatoes, peeled and sliced

2 medium red sweet potatoes, sliced

2 tablespoons olive oil

Salt and pepper to taste

Direction:

Preheat the air fryer to 3300F.

Place the grill pan accessory in the air fryer.

Take a large foil and place all ingredients in the middle. Give a good stir. Fold the foil and crimp the edges.

Place the foil on the grill pan.

Cook for 40 minutes.

Nutrition:

Calories: 362; Carbs: 68.4g; Protein: 6.3g; Fat: 9.4g

258. Grilled 'N Spiced Tomatoes On Garden Salad

Servings: 4

Cooking Time: 20 minutes

Ingredients

¼ cup golden raisings

¼ cup hazelnuts, toasted and chopped

¼ cup pistachios, toasted and chopped

½ cup chopped chives

¾ cup cilantro leaves, chopped

¾ cup fresh parsley, chopped

1 clove of garlic, minced

2 tablespoons white balsamic vinegar

3 large green tomatoes

4 leaves iceberg lettuce

5 tablespoons olive oil

Salt and pepper to taste

Direction:

Preheat the air fryer to 3300F.

Place the grill pan accessory in the air fryer.

In a mixing bowl, season the tomatoes with garlic, oil, salt and pepper to taste.

Place on the grill pan and grill for 20 minutes.

Once the tomatoes are done, toss in a salad bowl together with the rest of the Ingredients.

Nutrition:

Calories: 287; Carbs: 12.2g; Protein: 4.8g; Fat: 25.9g

259.Minty Green Beans With Shallots

Servings: 6

Cooking Time: 25 minutes

Ingredients

1 tablespoon fresh mint, chopped

1 tablespoon sesame seeds, toasted

1 tablespoon vegetable oil

1 teaspoon soy sauce

1-pound fresh green beans, trimmed

2 large shallots, sliced

2 tablespoons fresh basil, chopped

2 tablespoons pine nuts

Direction:

Preheat the air fryer to 3300F.

Place the grill pan accessory in the air fryer.

In a mixing bowl, combine the green beans, shallots, vegetable oil, and soy sauce.

Dump in the air fryer and cook for 25 minutes.

Once cooked, garnish with basil, mints, sesame seeds, and pine nuts.

Nutrition:

Calories per serving:307 ; Carbs: 11.2g; Protein: 23.7g; Fat: 19.7g

260. Vegie Grill Recipe With Tandoori Spice

Servings: 6

Cooking Time: 20 minutes

Ingredients

½ head cauliflower, cut into florets

½ cup yogurt

1 carrot,, peeled and shaved to 1/8-inch thick

1 cup young ears of corn

1 handful sugar snap peas

1 small zucchini, cut into thick slices

1 yellow sweet pepper, seeded and chopped

2 small onions, cut into wedges

2 tablespoons canola oil

2-inch fresh ginger, minced

3 tablespoons Tandoori spice blend

6 cloves of garlic, minced

Direction:

Preheat the air fryer to 3300F.

Place the grill pan accessory in the air fryer.

In a Ziploc bag, put all Ingredients: and give a shake to season all vegetables.

Dump all Ingredients: on the grill pan and cook for 20 minutes.

Make sure to give the vegetables a shake halfway through the cooking time.

Nutrition:

Calories per serving:126 ; Carbs: 17.9g; Protein: 2.9g; Fat: 6.1g

261. Creole Seasoned Vegetables

Servings: 5

Cooking Time: 15 minutes

Ingredients

¼ cup honey

¼ cup yellow mustard

1 large red bell pepper, sliced

1 teaspoon black pepper

1 teaspoon salt

2 large yellow squash, cut into ½ inch thick slices

2 medium zucchinis, cut into ½ inch thick slices

2 teaspoons creole seasoning

2 teaspoons smoked paprika

3 tablespoons olive oil

Direction:

Preheat the air fryer to 3300F.

Place the grill pan accessory in the air fryer.

In a Ziploc bag, put the zucchini, squash, red bell pepper, olive oil, salt and pepper. Give a shake to season all vegetables.

Place on the grill pan and cook for 15 minutes.

Meanwhile, prepare the sauce by combining the mustard, honey, paprika, and creole seasoning. Season with salt to taste.

Serve the vegetables with the sauce.

Nutrition:

Calories: 164; Carbs: 21.5g; Protein: 2.6g; Fat: 8.9g

262. Spicy Veggie Recipe From Thailand

Servings: 4

Cooking Time: 15 minutes

Ingredients

1 ½ cups packed cilantro leaves

1 tablespoon black pepper

1 tablespoon chili garlic sauce

1/3 cup vegetable oil

2 pounds vegetable of your choice, sliced into cubes

2 tablespoons fish sauce

8 cloves of garlic, minced

Direction:

Preheat the air fryer to 3300F.

Place the grill pan accessory in the air fryer.

Place all Ingredients: in a mixing bowl and toss to coat all Ingredients.

Put in the grill pan and cook for 15 minutes.

Nutrition:

Calories: 340; Carbs: 34.44g; Protein:8.8 g; Fat: 19.5g

263. Melted Cheese 'N Almonds On Tomato

Servings: 3

Cooking Time: 20 minutes

Ingredients

¼ cup toasted almonds

1 yellow red bell pepper, chopped

3 large tomatoes

4 ounces Monterey Jack cheese

Salt and pepper to taste

Direction:

Preheat the air fryer to 3300F.

Place the grill pan accessory in the air fryer.

Slice the tops of the tomatoes and remove the seeds to create hollow "cups."

In a mixing bowl, combine the cheese, bell pepper, and almonds. Season with salt and pepper to taste.

Stuff the tomatoes with the cheese filling.

Place the stuffed tomatoes on the grill pan and cook for 15 to 20 minutes.

Nutrition:

Calories: 125; Carbs: 13g; Protein: 10g; Fat: 14g

264. Hollandaise Topped Grilled Asparagus

Servings: 6

Cooking Time: 15 minutes

Ingredients

¼ teaspoon black pepper

½ cup butter, melted

½ lemon juice

½ teaspoon salt

½ teaspoon salt

1 teaspoon chopped tarragon leaves

2 tablespoons olive oil

3 egg yolks

3 pounds asparagus spears, trimmed

A pinch of mustard powder

A punch of ground white pepper

Direction:

Preheat the air fryer to 3300F.

Place the grill pan accessory in the air fryer.

In a Ziploc bag, combine the asparagus, olive oil, salt and pepper. Give a good shake to combine everything.

Dump on to the grill pan and cook for 15 minutes.

Meanwhile, on a double boiler over medium flame, whisk the egg yolks, lemon juice, and salt until silky. Add the mustard powder, white pepper and melted butter. Keep whisking until the sauce is smooth. Garnish with tarragon leaves.

Drizzle the sauce over asparagus spears.

Nutrition:

Calories: 253; Carbs: 10.2g; Protein: 6.7g; Fat: 22.4g

265. Garlic-Wine Flavored Vegetables

Servings: 4

Cooking Time: 15 minutes

Ingredients

¼ cup chopped fresh basil

1 ½ tablespoons honey1 teaspoon Dijon mustard

1 cup baby Portobello mushrooms, chopped

1 package frozen chopped vegetables

1 red onion, sliced

1/3 cup olive oil

3 tablespoon red wine vinegar

4 cloves of garlic, minced

Salt and pepper to taste

Direction:

Preheat the air fryer to 3300F.

Place the grill pan accessory in the air fryer.

In a Ziploc bag, combine the vegetables and season with salt, pepper, and garlic. Give a good shake to combine everything.

Dump on to the grill pan and cook for 15 minutes.

Meanwhile, combine the rest of the Ingredients: on bowl and season with more salt and pepper.

Drizzle the grilled vegetables with the sauce.

Nutrition:

Calories: 200; Carbs: 8.3g; Protein: 2.1g; Fat: 18.2g

266. Pepper-Pineapple With Butter-Sugar Glaze

Servings: 2

Cooking Time: 10 minutes

Ingredients

1 medium-sized pineapple, peeled and sliced

1 red bell pepper, seeded and julienned

1 teaspoon brown sugar

2 teaspoons melted butter

Salt to taste

Direction:

Preheat the air fryer to 3900F.

Place the grill pan accessory in the air fryer.

Mix all ingredients in a Ziploc bag and give a good shake.

Dump onto the grill pan and cook for 10 minutes making sure that you flip the pineapples every 5 minutes.

Nutrition:

Calories: 295; Carbs: 57g; Protein: 1g; Fat: 8g

Chapter 8 Desserts Recipes

267. Chocolate Cookies

Preparation Time: 10 minutes

Cooking time: 25 minutes

Servings: 12

Ingredients:

1 teaspoon vanilla extract

½ cup coconut butter, melted

1 tablespoon flax meal combined with 2 tablespoons water

4 tablespoons coconut sugar

2 cups flour

½ cup unsweetened vegan chocolate chips

Directions:

In a bowl, mix flax meal with vanilla extract and sugar and stir well.

Add melted butter, flour and half of the chocolate chips and stir everything.

Transfer this to a pan that fits your air fryer, spread the rest of the chocolate chips on top, introduce in the fryer at 330 degrees F and bake for 25 minutes.

Slice when it's cold and serve.

Enjoy!

Nutrition: calories 230, fat 12, fiber 2, carbs 13, protein 5

268. Simple And Sweet Bananas

Preparation Time: 10 minutes

Cooking time: 15 minutes

Servings: 4

Ingredients:

3 tablespoons coconut butter

2 tablespoons flax meal combined with 2 tablespoons water

8 bananas, peeled and halved

½ cup corn flour

3 tablespoons cinnamon powder

1 cup vegan breadcrumbs

Directions:

Heat up a pan with the butter over medium-high heat, add breadcrumbs, stir and cook for 4 minutes and then transfer to a bowl.

Roll each banana in flour, flax meal and breadcrumbs mix.

Arrange bananas in your air fryer's basket, dust with cinnamon sugar and cook at 280 degrees F for 10 minutes.

Transfer to plates and serve.

Enjoy!

Nutrition: calories 214, fat 1, fiber 4, carbs 12, protein 4

269. Coffee Pudding

Preparation Time: 10 minutes

Cooking time: 10 minutes

Servings: 4

Ingredients:

4 ounces coconut butter

4 ounces dark vegan chocolate, chopped

Juice of ½ orange

1 teaspoon baking powder

2 ounces whole wheat flour

½ teaspoon instant coffee

2 tablespoons flax meal combined with 2 tablespoons water

2 ounces coconut sugar

Directions:

Heat up a pan with the coconut butter over medium heat, add chocolate and orange juice, stir well and take off heat.

In a bowl, mix sugar with instant coffee and flax meal, beat using your mixer, add chocolate mix, flour, salt and baking powder and stir well.

Pour this into a greased pan, introduce in your air fryer, cook at 360 degrees F for 10 minutes, divide between plates and serve.

Enjoy!

Nutrition: calories 189, fat 6, fiber 4, carbs 14, protein 3

270. Almond And Vanilla Cake

Preparation Time: 10 minutes

Cooking time: 30 minutes

Servings: 8

Ingredients:

1 and ½ cup stevia

1 cup flour

¼ cup cocoa powder+ 2 tablespoons

½ cup chocolate almond milk

2 teaspoons baking powder

2 tablespoons canola oil

1 teaspoon vanilla extract

1 and ½ cups hot water

Cooking spray

Directions:

In a bowl, mix flour with 2 tablespoons cocoa, baking powder, almond milk, oil and vanilla extract, whisk well and spread on the bottom of a cake pan greased with cooking spray.

In a separate bowl, mix stevia with the rest of the cocoa and the water, whisk well and spread over the batter in the pan.

Introduce in the fryer and cook at 350 degrees F for 30 minutes.

Leave the cake to cool down, slice and serve.

Enjoy!

Nutrition: calories 250, fat 4, fiber 3, carbs 10, protein 2

271. Blueberry Cake

Preparation Time: 10 minutes

Cooking time: 30 minutes

Servings: 6

Ingredients:

½ cup whole wheat flour

¼ teaspoon baking powder

¼ teaspoon stevia

¼ cup blueberries

1/3 cup almond milk

1 teaspoon olive oil

1 teaspoon flaxseed, ground

½ teaspoon lemon zest, grated

¼ teaspoon vanilla extract

¼ teaspoon lemon extract

Cooking spray

Directions:

In a bowl, mix flour with baking powder, stevia, blueberries, milk, oil, flaxseeds, lemon zest, vanilla extract and lemon extract and whisk well.

Spray a cake pan with cooking spray, line it with parchment paper, pour cake batter, introduce in the fryer and cook at 350 degrees F for 30 minutes.

Leave the cake to cool down, slice and serve.

Enjoy!

Nutrition: calories 210, fat 4, fiber 4, carbs 10, protein 4

272. Peach Cobbler

Preparation Time: 10 minutes

Cooking time: 30 minutes

Servings: 4

Ingredients:

4 cups peaches, peeled and sliced

¼ cup coconut sugar

½ teaspoon cinnamon powder

1 and ½ cups vegan crackers, crushed

¼ cup stevia

¼ teaspoon nutmeg, ground

½ cup almond milk

1 teaspoon vanilla extract

Cooking spray

Directions:

In a bowl, mix peaches with coconut sugar and cinnamon and stir.

In a separate bowl, mix crackers with stevia, nutmeg, almond milk and vanilla extract and stir.

Spray a pie pan that fits your air fryer with cooking spray and spread peaches on the bottom.

Add crackers mix, spread, introduce into the fryer and cook at 350 degrees F for 30 minutes

Divide the cobbler between plates and serve.

Enjoy!

Nutrition: calories 201, fat 4, fiber 4, carbs 7, protein 3

273. Easy Pears Dessert

Preparation Time: 10 minutes

Cooking time: 25 minutes

Servings: 12

Ingredients:

6 big pears, cored and chopped

½ cup raisins

1 teaspoon ginger powder

¼ cup coconut sugar

1 teaspoon lemon zest, grated

Directions:

In a pan that fits your air fryer, mix pears with raisins, ginger, sugar and lemon zest, stir, introduce in the fryer and cook at 350 degrees F for 25 minutes.

Divide into bowls and serve cold.

Enjoy!

Nutrition: calories 200, fat 3, fiber 4, carbs 6, protein 6

274. Sweet Strawberry Mix

Preparation Time: 10 minutes

Cooking time: 20 minutes

Servings: 10

Ingredients:

2 tablespoons lemon juice

2 pounds strawberries

4 cups coconut sugar

1 teaspoon cinnamon powder

1 teaspoon vanilla extract

Directions:

In a pan that fits your air fryer, mix strawberries with coconut sugar, lemon juice, cinnamon and vanilla, stir gently, introduce in the fryer and cook at 350 degrees F for 20 minutes

Divide into bowls and serve cold.

Enjoy!

Nutrition: calories 140, fat 0, fiber 1, carbs 5, protein 2

275. Sweet Bananas And Sauce

Preparation Time: 10 minutes

Cooking time: 20 minutes

Servings: 4

Ingredients:

Juice of ½ lemon

3 tablespoons agave nectar

1 tablespoon coconut oil

4 bananas, peeled and sliced diagonally

½ teaspoon cardamom seeds

Directions:

Arrange bananas in a pan that fits your air fryer, add agave nectar, lemon juice, oil and cardamom, introduce in the fryer and cook at 360 degrees F for 20 minutes

Divide bananas and sauce between plates and serve.

Enjoy!

Nutrition: calories 210, fat 1, fiber 2, carbs 8, protein 3

276. Orange Cake

Preparation Time: 10 minutes

Cooking time: 30 minutes

Servings: 4

Ingredients:

Cooking spray

1 teaspoon baking powder

1 cup almond flour

1 cup coconut sugar

½ teaspoon cinnamon powder

3 tablespoons coconut oil, melted

½ cup almond milk

½ cup pecans, chopped

¾ cup water

½ cup raisins

½ cup orange peel, grated

¾ cup orange juice

Directions:

In a bowl, mix flour with half of the sugar, baking powder, cinnamon, 2 tablespoons oil, milk, pecans and raisins, stir and pour this in a greased cake pan that fits your air fryer.

Heat up a small pan over medium heat, add water, orange juice, orange peel, the rest of the oil and the rest of the sugar, stir, bring to a boil, pour over the mix from the pan, introduce in the fryer and cook at 330 degrees F for 30 minutes.

Serve cold.

Enjoy!

Nutrition: calories 282, fat 3, fiber 1, carbs 4, protein 3

277. Stuffed Apples

Preparation Time: 10 minutes

Cooking time: 25 minutes

Servings: 5

Ingredients:

5 apples, tops cut off and cored

5 figs

1/3 cup coconut sugar

¼ cup pecans, chopped

2 teaspoons lemon zest, grated

½ teaspoon cinnamon powder

1 tablespoon lemon juice

1tablespoon coconut oil

Directions:

In a bowl mix figs, coconut sugar, pecans, lemon zest, cinnamon, lemon juice and coconut oil and stir.

Stuff the apples with this mix, introduce them in your air fryer and cook at 365 degrees F for 25 minutes.

Enjoy!

Nutrition: calories 200, fat 1, fiber 2, carbs 6, protein 3

278. Apples And Mandarin Sauce

Preparation Time: 10 minutes

Cooking time: 20 minutes

Servings: 4

Ingredients:

4 apples, cored, peeled and cored

2 cups mandarin juice

¼ cup maple syrup

2 teaspoons cinnamon powder

1 tablespoon ginger, grated

Directions:

In a pan that fits your air fryer, mix apples with mandarin juice, maple syrup, cinnamon and ginger, introduce in the fryer and cook at 365 degrees F for 20 minutes

Divide apples mix between plates and serve warm.

Enjoy!

Nutrition: calories 170, fat 1, fiber 2, carbs 6, protein 4

279. Almond Cookies

Preparation Time: 10 minutes

Cooking time: 30 minutes

Servings: 12

Ingredients:

1 tablespoon flaxseed mixed with 2 tablespoons water

¼ cup coconut oil, melted

1 cup coconut sugar

½ teaspoon vanilla extract

1 teaspoon baking powder

1 and ½ cups almond meal

½ cup almonds, chopped

Directions:

In a bowl, mix oil with sugar, vanilla extract and flax meal and whisk.

Add baking powder, almond meal and almonds and stir well.

Spread cookie mix on a lined baking sheet, introduce in your air fryer and cook at 340 degrees F for 30 minutes.

Leave cookie sheet to cool down, cut into medium pieces and serve.

Enjoy!

Nutrition: calories 210, fat 2, fiber 1, carbs 7, protein 6

280. Easy Pumpkin Cake

Preparation Time: 10 minutes

Cooking time: 40 minutes

Servings: 10

Ingredients:

1 and ½ teaspoons baking powder

Cooking spray

1 cup pumpkin puree

2 cups almond flour

½ teaspoon baking soda

1 and ½ teaspoons cinnamon, ground

¼ teaspoon ginger, ground

1 tablespoon coconut oil, melted

1 tablespoon flaxseed mixed with 2 tablespoons water

1 tablespoon vanilla extract

1/3 cup maple syrup

1 teaspoon lemon juice

Directions:

In a bowl, flour with baking powder, baking soda, cinnamon and ginger and stir.

Add flaxseed, coconut oil, vanilla, pumpkin puree, maple syrup and lemon juice, stir and pour into a greased cake pan.

Introduce in your air fryer, cook at 330 degrees F for 40 minutes, leave aside to cool down, slice and serve.

Enjoy!

Nutrition: calories 202, fat 3, fiber 2, carbs 6, protein 1

281. Sweet Potato Mix

Preparation Time: 10 minutes

Cooking time: 30 minutes

Servings: 8

Ingredients:

1 cup water

1 tablespoon lemon peel, grated

½ cup coconut sugar

3 sweet potatoes peeled and sliced

¼ cup cashew butter

¼ cup maple syrup

1 cup pecans, chopped

Directions:

In a pan that fits your air fryer, mix water with lemon peel, coconut sugar, potatoes, cashew butter, maple syrup and pecans, stir, introduce in the fryer and cook at 350 degrees F for 30 minutes

Divide sweet potato pudding into bowls and serve cold.

Enjoy!

Nutrition: calories 210, fat 4, fiber 3, carbs 10, protein 4

282. Cinnamon Rice

Preparation Time: 10 minutes

Cooking time: 35 minutes

Servings: 4

Ingredients:

3 and ½ cups water

1 cup coconut sugar

2 cups white rice, washed and rinsed

2 cinnamon sticks

½ cup coconut, shredded

Directions:

In your air fryer, mix water with coconut sugar, rice, cinnamon and coconut, stir, cover and cook at 365 degrees F for 35 minutes.

Divide pudding into cups and serve cold.

Enjoy!

Nutrition: calories 213, fat 4, fiber 6, carbs 9, protein 4

283. Cranberry Pudding

Preparation Time: 10 minutes

Cooking time: 30 minutes

Servings: 4

Ingredients:

4 ounces dried cranberries, chopped

A drizzle of olive oil

4 ounces dried apricots, chopped

1 cup white flour

3 teaspoons baking powder

1 cup coconut sugar

1 teaspoon ginger powder

A pinch of cinnamon powder

15 tablespoons coconut butter

3 tablespoons maple syrup

3 tablespoons flax meal mixed with 3 tablespoons water

1 carrot, grated

Directions:

Grease a heatproof pudding pan with a drizzle of oil.

In a blender, mix flour with baking powder, sugar, cinnamon, ginger, butter, maple syrup and flax meal and pulse well.

Add dried fruits and carrot, fold them into the batter and spread this mix into the pudding mold.

Put the pudding in your air fryer and cook at 365 degrees F for 30 minutes.

Leave the pudding aside to cool down, slice and serve.

Enjoy!

Nutrition: calories 262, fat 7, fiber 4, carbs 12, protein 4

284. Chocolate And Coconut Bars

Preparation Time: 10 minutes

Cooking time: 7 minutes

Servings: 12

Ingredients:

1 cup sugar free and vegan chocolate chips

2 tablespoons coconut butter

2/3 cup coconut cream

2 tablespoons stevia

¼ teaspoon vanilla extract

Directions:

Put the cream in a bowl, add stevia, butter and chocolate chips and stir

Leave aside for 5 minutes, stir well and mix the vanilla.

Transfer the mix into a lined baking sheet, introduce in your air fryer and cook at 356 degrees F for 7 minutes.

Leave the mix aside to cool down, slice and serve.

Enjoy!

Nutrition: calories 120, fat 5, fiber 4, carbs 6, protein 1

285. Raspberry Bars

Preparation Time: 10 minutes

Cooking time: 6 minutes

Servings: 12

Ingredients:

½ cup coconut butter, melted

½ cup coconut oil

½ cup raspberries, dried

¼ cup swerve

½ cup coconut, shredded

Directions:

In your food processor, blend dried berries very well.

In a bowl that fits your air fryer, mix oil with butter, swerve, coconut and raspberries, toss well, introduce in the fryer and cook at 320 degrees F for 6 minutes.

Spread this on a lined baking sheet, keep in the fridge for an hour, slice and serve.

Enjoy!

Nutrition: calories 164, fat 22, fiber 2, carbs 4, protein 2

286. Vanilla And Blueberry Squares

Preparation Time: 10 minutes

Cooking time: 20 minutes

Servings: 8

Ingredients:

5 ounces coconut oil, melted

½ teaspoon baking powder

4 tablespoons stevia

1 teaspoon vanilla

4 ounces coconut cream

3 tablespoons flax meal combined with 3 tablespoons water

½ cup blueberries

Directions:

In a bowl, mix coconut oil with flax meal, coconut cream, vanilla, stevia and baking powder and blend using an immersion blender.

Fold blueberries, pour everything into a square baking dish that fits your air fryer, introduce in the fryer and cook at 320 degrees F for 20 minutes.

Slice into squares and serve cold.

Enjoy!

Nutrition: calories 150, fat 2, fiber 3, carbs 6, protein 4

287. Cocoa Brownies

Preparation Time: 10 minutes

Cooking time: 20 minutes

Servings: 12

Ingredients:

6 ounces coconut oil, melted

3 tablespoons flax meal combined with 3 tablespoons water

3 ounces cocoa powder

2 teaspoons vanilla

½ teaspoon baking powder

4 ounces coconut cream

5 tablespoons stevia

Directions:

In a blender, mix flax meal with oil, cocoa powder, baking powder, vanilla, cream and stevia and stir using a mixer.

Pour this into a lined baking dish that fits your air fryer, introduce in the fryer and cook at 350 degrees F for 20 minutes.

Slice into rectangles and serve cold

Enjoy!

Nutrition: calories 208, fat 14, fiber 2, carbs 13, protein 5

288. Easy Blackberries Scones

Preparation Time: 10 minutes

Cooking time: 10 minutes

Servings: 10

Ingredients:

½ cup coconut flour

1 cup blackberries

2 tablespoons flax meal combined with 2 tablespoons water

½ cup coconut cream

½ cup coconut butter

½ cup almond flour

5 tablespoons stevia

2 teaspoons vanilla extract

2 teaspoons baking powder

Directions:

In a bowl, mix almond flour with coconut flour, baking powder and blackberries and stir well.

In another bowl, mix cream with butter, vanilla extract, stevia and flax meal and stir well.

Combine the 2 mixtures, stir until you obtain your dough, shape 10 triangles from this mix, place them on a lined baking sheet, introduce in the air fryer and cook at 350 degrees F for 10 minutes.

Serve them cold.

Enjoy!

Nutrition: calories 170, fat 2, fiber 2, carbs 4, protein 3

289. Easy Buns

Preparation Time: 10 minutes

Cooking time: 30 minutes

Servings: 8

Ingredients:

½ cup coconut flour

1/3 cup psyllium husks

2 tablespoons stevia

1 teaspoon baking powder

½ teaspoon cinnamon powder

½ teaspoon cloves, ground

3 tablespoons flax meal combined with 3 tablespoons water

Some chocolate chips, unsweetened

Directions:

In a bowl, mix flour with psyllium husks, swerve, baking powder, salt, cinnamon, cloves and chocolate chips and stir well.

Add water and flax meal, stir well until you obtain a dough, shape 8 buns and arrange them on a lined baking sheet.

Introduce in the air fryer and cook at 350 degrees for 30 minutes.

Serve these buns warm.

Nutrition: calories 140, fat 3, fiber 3, carbs 7, protein 6

290. Lemon Cream

Preparation Time: 10 minutes

Cooking time: 30 minutes

Servings: 6

Ingredients:

1 and 1/3 pint almond milk

1 medium banana

4 tablespoons lemon zest, grated

3 tablespoons flax meal combined with 3 tablespoons water

5 tablespoons stevia

2 tablespoons lemon juice

Directions:

In a bowl, mix mashed banana with milk and swerve and stir very well.

Add lemon zest and lemon juice, whisk well, pour into ramekins, place them in your air fryer, cook at 360 degrees F for 30 minutes and serve cold.

Enjoy!

Nutrition: calories 180, fat 6, fiber 2, carbs 5, protein 7

291. Cocoa Berries Cream

Preparation Time: 10 minutes

Cooking time: 10 minutes

Servings: 4

Ingredients:

3 tablespoons cocoa powder

14 ounces coconut cream

1 cup blackberries

1 cup raspberries

2 tablespoons stevia

Directions:

In a bowl, whisk cocoa powder with stevia and cream and stir.

Add raspberries and blackberries, toss gently, transfer to a pan that fits your air fryer, introduce in the fryer and cook at 350 degrees F for 10 minutes.

Divide into bowls and serve cold.

Enjoy!

Nutrition: calories 205, fat 34, fiber 2, carbs 6, protein 2

292. Apple Chips

Preparation Time: 10 minutes

Cooking Time: 20 minutes

Servings: 2

Ingredients:

1 apple, sliced thinly

Salt to taste

¼ teaspoon ground cinnamon

Method:

Preheat the air fryer to 350 degrees F.

Toss the apple slices in salt and cinnamon.

Add to the air fryer.

Let cool before serving.

Nutrition:

Calories 59

Total Fat 0.2g

Saturated Fat 0g

Cholesterol 0mg

Sodium 79mg

Total Carbohydrate 15.6g

Dietary Fiber 2.9g

Total Sugars 11.6g

Protein 0.3g

Potassium 121mg

293. Fruit Crumble

Preparation Time: 10 minutes

Cooking Time: 15 minutes

Servings: 4

Ingredients:

1 apple, diced

¼ cup frozen blueberries

¼ cup frozen strawberries

¼ cup and 1 tablespoon brown rice flour

2 tablespoons sugar

½ teaspoon ground cinnamon

2 tablespoons vegan butter

Method:

Preheat your air fryer to 350 degrees F.

In a ramekin, combine the apple, blueberries and strawberries.

In another bowl, mix the rest of the ingredients.

Serve this mixture over the fruit mix.

Cook at 350 degrees F for 15 minutes.

Nutrition:

Calories 310

Total Fat 12 g

Saturated Fat 7 g

Cholesterol 31 mg

Sodium 5 mg

Total Carbohydrate 50 g

Dietary Fiber 5 g

Total Sugars 26 g

Protein 2 g

Potassium 557 mg

294. Fruit Kebab

Preparation Time: 30 minutes

Cooking Time: 6 minutes

Servings: 10

Ingredients:

1 teaspoon maple syrup

1 teaspoon lemon juice

1 apple, diced

1 mango, diced

1 pear, diced

Salt to taste

Lemon zest

Method:

In a bowl, combine maple syrup and lemon juice.

Coat the fruit cubes with the mixture.

Season with salt.

Arrange in skewers.

Place the skewers inside the air fryer and cook at 360 degrees for 5 minutes.

Garnish with lemon zest.

Nutrition:

Calories 52

Total Fat 0.2g

Saturated Fat 0.1g

Cholesterol 0mg

Sodium 20mg

Total Carbohydrate 13.4g

Dietary Fiber 1.9g

Total Sugars 10.8g

Protein 0.5g

Potassium 123mg

295. Baked Apples With Pumpkin Spice

Preparation Time: 10 minutes

Cooking Time: 15 minutes

Servings: 4

Ingredients:

4 apples, sliced

¼ cup maple syrup

¼ cup rolled oats

¼ cup pecans, chopped

2 tablespoons raisins

1 teaspoon pumpkin spice seasoning

2/3 cup water

Method:

Coat apple slices with maple syrup and mix with oats, pecans and raisins.

Season with pumpkin spice.

Transfer the mixture into a small heatproof dish that can fit inside the air fryer.

In the air fryer, add the water.

Put the dish inside.

Cook at 340 degrees F for 15 minutes.

Nutrition:

Calories 206

Total Fat 1.4g

Saturated Fat 0.1g

Cholesterol 0mg

Sodium 6mg

Total Carbohydrate 51.2g

Dietary Fiber 6.2g

Total Sugars 37.7g

Protein 1.5g

Potassium 335mg

296. Vegan Brownies

Preparation Time: 15 minutes

Cooking Time: 20 minutes

Servings: 4

Ingredients:

½ cup whole wheat pastry flour

¼ cup cocoa powder

½ cup sugar

1 tablespoon ground flax seeds

¼ teaspoon salt

¼ cup almond milk

¼ cup aquafaba

½ teaspoon vanilla extract

Chopped walnuts

Cooking spray

Method:

Combine first five ingredients in a bowl.

Mix the rest of the ingredients except the walnuts in another bowl.

Slowly combine the two bowls.

Preheat your air fryer to 350 degrees F.

Spray air fryer with oil.

Pour the mixture into a heatproof pan.

Sprinkle top with walnuts.

Cook in the air fryer for 20 minutes.

Nutrition:

Calories 206

Total Fat 5.1g

Saturated Fat 3.7g

Cholesterol 0mg

Sodium 151mg

Total Carbohydrate 40.4g

Dietary Fiber 3.9g

Total Sugars 25.7g

Protein 3.1g

Potassium 189mg

297. Berry Crumble

Preparation Time: 15 minutes

Cooking Time: 12 minutes

Servings: 4

Ingredients:

½ cup blackberries

½ cup strawberries

1 cup blueberries

¼ cup flour

¼ cup sugar

1 teaspoon vanilla

½ cup quick oats

¼ cup brown sugar

1 teaspoon lemon juice

3 tablespoons melted butter

Method:

In a bowl, combine the berries, lemon juice and sugar.

In another bowl, mix the rest of the ingredients.

Toss the berries in the mixture.

Spray air fryer with oil.

Cook at 390 degrees F for 12 minutes.

Nutrition:

Calories 262

Total Fat 9.7g

Saturated Fat 5.6g

Cholesterol 23mg

Sodium 66mg

Total Carbohydrate 42.8g

Dietary Fiber 3.4g

Total Sugars 26.9g

Protein 2.9g

Potassium 148mg

298. Sweetened Plantains

Preparation Time: 5 minutes

Cooking Time: 8 minutes

Servings: 4

Ingredients:

2 ripe plantains, sliced

2 teaspoons avocado oil

Salt to taste

Maple syrup

Method:

Toss the plantains in oil.

Season with salt.

Cook in the air fryer basket at 400 degrees F for 10 minutes, shaking after 5 minutes.

Drizzle with maple syrup before serving.

Nutrition:

Calories 125

Total Fat 0.6g

Saturated Fat 0.2g

Cholesterol 0mg

Sodium 43mg

Total Carbohydrate 32g

Dietary Fiber 2.2g

Total Sugars 16.4g

Protein 1.2g

Potassium 464mg

299. Carrot Cake

Preparation Time: 10 minutes

Cooking Time: 15 minutes

Serving: 1

Ingredients:

Cooking spray

¼ cups whole wheat pastry flour

¼ teaspoon baking powder

1 tablespoon coconut sugar

1/8 teaspoon ground dried ginger

¼ teaspoon ground cinnamon

Salt to taste

2 tablespoons almond milk

2 teaspoons oil

2 tablespoons carrot, grated

1 tablespoons date, chopped

2 tablespoons walnuts, chopped

Water

Method:

Spray a heatproof mug with oil.

In a bowl, mix the flour, baking powder, sugar, ginger, cinnamon and salt.

Pour in the milk and oil.

Add the carrot, dates and walnuts.

Mix well.

Put the mug inside the air fryer.

Pour water around it.

Cook in the air fryer at 350 degrees for 15 minutes or until middle part is fully cooked.

Nutrition:

Calories 365

Total Fat 17.5g

Saturated Fat 6.9g

Cholesterol 0mg

Sodium 171mg

Total Carbohydrate 48g

Dietary Fiber 6.3g

Total Sugars 20.9g

Protein 7.8g

Potassium 406mg

300. Roasted Bananas

Preparation Time: 5 minutes

Cooking Time: 5 minutes

Servings: 2

Ingredients:

2 cups bananas, cubed

1 teaspoon avocado oil

1 tablespoon maple syrup

1 teaspoon brown sugar

1 cup almond milk

Method:

Coat the banana cubes with oil and maple syrup.

Sprinkle with brown sugar.

Cook in the air fryer at 375 degrees F for 5 minutes.

Drizzle milk on top of the bananas before serving.

Nutrition:

Calories 107

Total Fat 0.7g

Saturated Fat 0.0g

Cholesterol 0mg

Sodium 1mg

Total Carbohydrates 27g

Dietary Fiber 3.1g

Protein 1.3g

Sugars 14g

Potassium 422mg

301. Pear Crisp

Preparation Time: 10 minutes

Cooking Time: 25 minutes

Servings: 2

Ingredients:

1 cup flour

1 stick vegan butter

1 tablespoon cinnamon

½ cup sugar

2 pears, cubed

Method:

Mix flour and butter to form crumbly texture.

Add cinnamon and sugar.

Put the pears in the air fryer.

Pour and spread the mixture on top of the pears.

Cook at 350 degrees F for 25 minutes.

Nutrition:

Calories 544

Total Fat 0.9g

Saturated Fat 0.1g

Cholesterol 0mg

Sodium 4mg

Total Carbohydrate 132.3g

Dietary Fiber 10g

Total Sugars 70.6g

Protein 7.4g

Potassium 324mg

Conclusion

Becoming a vegan certainly has many benefits.

It's not easy at first but once you get used to it, you'll definitely reap its countless benefits, particularly for one's health.

It's good to know that there are modern appliances like the air fryer that can help make things easier for you when you make the transition.

Cheers to a healthier you! Good luck!

302. Small Batch Brownies

Servings: 4

Preparation Time: 10 mins

Cooking Time: 20 mins

Ingredients:

For the Dry Ingredients:

½ cup whole-wheat, gluten-free pastry flour

1 tbsp. ground flax seeds

¼ cup cocoa powder

½ cup vegan sugar

¼ tsp. salt

Wet Ingredients:

¼ cup almond milk

½ tsp. pure vanilla extract

¼ cup aquafaba

Extras:

¼ cup of: hazelnuts, chopped walnuts, pecans, shredded coconut, mini vegan chocolate chips

Directions:

Mix all the dry ingredients in one bowl.

In a Pyrex jug, mix all the wet and set aside.

Add the wet ingredients to the dry and mix to combine.

Add in the extra ingredients of your choice and mix again.

Preheat the air fryer to 350 degrees Fahrenheit.

Line a 5-inch cake tin with baking parchment paper if you want an oil-free recipe or spray the cake tin lightly with cooking oil spray if the recipe is not oil-free.

Place the pan in the air fryer basket.

Cook the brownies for 20 minutes. If the brownies are not done cook for 5 minutes more and repeat as needed. A cake tester inserted should come out relatively clean.

Recipe Notes:

Cooking times may vary depending on the size of the cake tin and the brand of air fryer used.

Nutrition:

Total Calories: 225.3 kcal.

Carbohydrates: 41g (Dietary Fiber: 4.8g, Sugar: 25g), Protein: 4g, Fat: 6.8g, Potassium: 169mg, Sodium: 157.8mg, Calcium: 3.5%, Vitamin A: 0.6%, Iron: 8.1%.

303. 2. Carrot Mug Cakes

Servings: 1

Preparation Time: 5 mins

Cooking Time: 15 mins

Ingredients:

¼ cups whole-wheat, gluten-free pastry flour,

1 tbsp. brown sugar or coconut sugar

¼ teaspoon ground cinnamon

¼ teaspoon baking powder

2 tbsp. almond milk plus 2 tsp. more

1 tbsp. raisins or chopped dates

2 tbsp. grated carrot

2 tbsp. chopped walnuts

1/8 teaspoon ground dried ginger

A pinch ground allspice

A pinch of salt

2 tsp. flavorless oil

Directions:

Lightly oil an oven-safe ceramic mug.

Add the flour, baking powder, sugar, ginger, allspice, cinnamon and salt then mix well with a fork.

Next add the carrot, milk, walnuts, raisins and oil and then mix again.

Bake in an air fryer at 350 degrees Fahrenheit for 15 minutes.

Check with a cake tester to make sure the middle is cooked.

If not, cook for 5 additional minutes.

Serve warm!

304.3. Beignets

Servings: 24

Preparation Time: 1 hr.

Cooking Time: 15 mins

Ingredients:

To make the powdered baking blend:

1 cup baking blend

1 tsp. organic corn starch

For the proofing:

1 cup full-fat coconut milk

1½ tsp. active baking yeast

3 tbsp. powdered baking blend

For the dough:

3 cups unbleached white flour

2 tbsp. aquafaba

2 tbsp. melted coconut oil

2 tsp. pure vanilla extract

Directions:

Add the corn starch and baking blend to a blender and blend until powdery smooth.

Gently heat the coconut milk until it's warm, at blood heat temperature.

Add the coconut milk to a mixer with the sugar and yeast. Let sit for 10 minutes, until the yeast starts foaming.

Using the paddle attachment, mix in the aquafaba, coconut oil and vanilla. Then add the flour one cup at a time.

Once the flour mixed in and the dough is coming away from the sides of the bowl of the mixer, change to a dough hook attachment.

Knead the dough in the mixer for about 3 minutes. The dough will be wetter than if making bread.

Place the dough in a mixing bowl and cover with a clean dish towel to rise for 1 hour.

Sprinkle some flour over a large clean cutting board and pat out the dough into a rectangle about ⅓ inch thick.

Cut into 24 squares and let prove for 30 minutes before cooking.

Preheat the air fryer to 390 degrees Fahrenheit. Cook the beignet in batches, so they cook evenly.

Cook for 3 minutes on one side and then flip over and then cook another 2 minutes.

Sprinkle with the powdered baking blend and enjoy!

305.4. Sweet Potato Dessert Fries

Servings: 4

Preparation Time: 5 mins

Cooking Time: 20 mins

Ingredients:

2 medium sweet potatoes, peeled

½ tbsp. coconut oil.

2 tsp. melted butter (for coating)

¼ cup coconut sugar or raw sugar

1 tbsp. arrowroot or cornstarch

1 - 2 tbsp. cinnamon

Icing sugar for dusting

Dipping Sauces:

Maple Frosting

Dessert Hummus

Honey or vanilla Greek yogurt

Directions:

Peel the sweet potatoes, wash with clean water and then pat dry.

Slice the sweet potatoes lengthways, about half an inch thick.

Toss the sweet potato slices in half a tablespoon of coconut oil and arrowroot or cornstarch.

Place in the fries into the air fryer at 370 degrees Fahrenheit for 18 minutes. Shake halfway through cooking to ensure they cook evenly.

Remove the fries from the air fryer and place in a bowl. Drizzle 2 tea spoons (optional) of butter on top of fries.

Mix in the cinnamon and sugar and toss together with the fries

Place on a serving plate and serve, garnished with powdered sugar.

Serve the fries with the dipping sauce of your choice.

These fries should keep, refrigerated and wrapped in aluminum foil, for 2 – 3 days.

Nutrition:

Calories: 130 kcal.

Total Carbohydrate 26.9g (Dietary Fiber 3g, Sugars 14.8g), Protein 1.2g, Total Fat 2.3g (Saturated Fat 1.7), Cholesterol 1.3mg, Sodium 45.5mg

306.5. Pumpkin Baked Apples

Servings: 4

Preparation Time: 10 mins

Cooking Time: 15 mins

Ingredients:

For the Baked Apples:

4 Gala or Fuji apples

⅓ cup rolled oats

⅔ cup water

¼ cup maple syrup

1 tsp. pumpkin spice seasoning

2 tbsp. raisins

¼ cup chopped pecans

Directions:

Core the apples, but don't cut through to the bottom. Cut at a slight angle, to form a sort of a cone of apple core from the center.

In a small bowl, mix together all the ingredients for the baked apples, except for the water.

Pour the water into a shallow, ceramic ovenproof dish that fits the air fryer basket.

Arrange the apples in the dish in a single layer.

Cook at 340 degrees Fahrenheit for 15 minutes, or until the apples are tender when pierced. You can continue cooking for another 2-3 minutes if they're not done, and check on them again.

Serve warm, at room temperature, or cold if desired.

Recipe Notes:

Use tongs to gently remove the apples from the air fryer basket.

307.6. Strawberry Lemonade Pop Tart

Servings: 14 pop tarts

Preparation Time: 40 mins

Cooking Time: 10 mins

Ingredients:

For the Strawberry Chia Jam:

3 cups sliced strawberries, frozen or fresh

3 tbsp. chia seeds

2 tsp. maple syrup, or to taste

2 tbsp. lemon juice, or to taste

For the Pop-tarts:

1 cup all-purpose flour

1 cup whole-wheat pastry flour

2 tbsp. light brown sugar

¼ tsp. salt

½ cup ice cold water

⅔ cup very cold coconut oil

½ tsp. vanilla extract

For the Lemon Glaze:

1¼ cup powdered sugar

Zest of 1 lemon

2 tbsp. lemon juice

¼ tsp. vanilla extract

1 tsp. melted coconut oil

Colorful sprinkles for decoration

Directions:

To make the Chia Jam:

In a sauce pan, heat the strawberries and cherries until they start to get syrupy and give out their juice.

Once they are super soft, mash them until the mixture is jammy, and still with some visible bits of fruit.

Add in the maple syrup and lemon juice Adjust the lemon and maple syrup depending on the level of sweetness in the fruit.

Take the mixture off the heat, transfer it to a glass container and add in the chia seeds.

Allow the mixture to set for 20 minutes. It will thicken on standing.

To make the Pop-tarts:

In a large bowl, mix both flours, sugar and salt.

Cut in the cold coconut oil with a fork or pastry cutter until the mixture resembles tiny peas.

Add the vanilla extract and slowly add in the ice cold water.

It should be moist enough to form it into a ball without flaking away, but not too sticky either.

Cut the dough in half and flour a work surface and rolling pin.

Roll out the dough to just a few millimeters thick then cut into 7 cm by 5 cm rectangles.

Place the rectangles on a baking sheet lined with a silicone baking sheet or parchment paper.

Place a heaping teaspoon of jam onto half of the dough rectangles. Moisten all around the perimeter of the dough.

Top with another dough rectangle, and crimp the edges with a fork to seal.

Poke three sets of three holes into the top of the pop tart with your fork. Place pop tarts on the baking sheet in the fridge to set for 20 minutes.

Heat the air fryer to 400 degrees Fahrenheit.

Add four pop-tarts to the air fryer basket and cook for 10 minutes.

Remove and repeat with the remaining pop-tarts until they're all cooked. Cool for 20 minutes before serving.

To make the Lemon Glaze:

In a bowl, mix together the icing sugar, lemon juice, coconut oil, vanilla extract and lemon zest.

Drizzle the icing on each of the pop-tarts and decorate with sprinkles. Let the icing set and enjoy!

308.7. Blueberry Apple Crumble

Servings: 2

Preparation Time: 5 mins

Cooking Time: 15 mins

Ingredients:

1 apple, finely diced

¼ cup brown rice flour plus 1 tbsp. more

½ cup frozen strawberries, blueberries or peaches

2 tbsp. nondairy butter

2 tbsp. sugar

½ tsp. ground cinnamon

Directions:

Preheat the air fryer to 350 degrees Fahrenheit for 5 minutes.

Combine the apple and frozen berries or peaches in an air fryer–safe baking pan.

In a small bowl, combine the flour, cinnamon, sugar, and butter.

Spoon the crumble mixture over the fruit. Sprinkle a little extra flour all the fruit to cover any that are exposed.

Cook at 350 degrees Fahrenheit for 15 minutes.

Serve warm with dairy-free whipped cream or ice cream

309.8. Apple, Strawberries And Peaches Crumble

Servings: 2

Preparation Time: 5 mins

Cooking Time: 15 mins

Ingredients:

1 apple, finely diced

¼ cup brown rice flour plus 1 tbsp. more

½ cup frozen strawberries, blueberries or peaches

2 tbsp. nondairy butter

2 tbsp. sugar

½ tsp. ground cinnamon

Directions:

Preheat the air fryer to 350 degrees Fahrenheit for 5 minutes.

Combine the apple and frozen berries or peaches in an air fryer–safe baking pan.

In a small bowl, combine the flour, cinnamon, sugar, and butter.

Spoon the crumble mixture over the fruit. Sprinkle a little extra flour all the fruit to cover any that are exposed.

Cook at 350 degrees Fahrenheit for 15 minutes.

Serve warm with dairy-free whipped cream or ice cream

310.9. Cinnamon Pears

Servings: 2-4

Preparation Time: 5 mins

Cooking Time: 10 mins

Ingredients:

2 unripe pears, peeled, cored, cut in half

2 tbsp. vegan butter

1 tsp. pure vanilla extract

½ tsp. cinnamon

To Garnish:

Sprinkle of nutmeg

Directions:

Preheat the air fryer to 350 degrees Fahrenheit.

Melt the butter and add to it the vanilla extract and cinnamon, mixing well.

Baste the cut sides of the pears with the butter and place them cut side down into a baking pan that fits the air fryer.

Baste the top of the pears and bake at 350 degrees Fahrenheit for 10 minutes.

Flip the pears over and baste again.

Bake for 2 more minutes at the same temperature.

Give the pears a final baste and set on to serving plates.

Serve hot with whipped cream or ice cream.

311. Churro Doughnuts

Servings: 6

Preparation Time: 1 hr. 15 mins

Cooking Time: 6 mins

Ingredients:

1 cup white all-purpose flour

1 tsp. baking powder

¼ cup organic sugar

¼ tsp. ground cinnamon

½ tsp. salt

2 tbsp. aquafaba

¼ cup soy or almond milk

1 tbsp. melted coconut oil

2 tsp. ground cinnamon

2 tbsp. sugar

Directions:

In a large bowl, combine the flour, baking powder, sugar, cinnamon and salt. Mix well to combine.

Add the coconut oil, aquafaba, and soy milk and combine.

When the dough is ready, it should be a ball of slightly sticky dough.

Stick the dough in the refrigerator for at least 1 hour.

In a shallow bowl, mix together the cinnamon and the 2 tablespoons of sugar. Set this cinnamon-sugar aside.

Cut a piece of baking parchment paper so it covers some of the bottom of the air fryer.

Remove the dough from the fridge, and knead.

Divide into 12 pieces, forming them into balls.

Dredge each ball in cinnamon sugar, and put into a single layer on the baking parchment paper, leaving at least 1 inch around each ball.

Air fry at 370 degrees Fahrenheit for 6 minutes. Do not shake the churro balls.

Let the doughnuts cool for 5-10 minutes before removing from the basket.

Serve hot with chocolate sauce.

312. Berry Cake

Servings: 6

Preparation Time: 10 mins

Cooking Time: 20 mins

Ingredients:

1½ cup whole meal self-raising unbleached flour

⅔ cup xylitol

¾ cup soy milk – 3/4 cup

1 tsp. white vinegar

1 tbsp. vegetable oil

1 tsp. lemon zest

⅔ - ¾ cup mixed berries

Directions:

Lightly coat a 6-inch cake pan with cooking oil spray.

Mix the oil and xylitol in one jug and then whisk the soy milk and vinegar in a separate jug. Set aside to curdle.

Combine all the above mixtures and add the lemon zest, oil and berries.

Fold in the self-raising flour and mix well.

Pour the batter into the oiled cake pan and tap lightly to settle the batter.

Bake in the air fryer at 175 degrees Celsius for 18 – 20 minutes.

313. Banana Bread

Banana bread made in the air fryer are so healthy, delicious and easy to make. Perfect for breakfast or as an afternoon snack, and even better ready in under 30 minutes.

Servings: 1

Preparation Time: 10 mins

Cooking Time: 20 mins

Ingredients:

2 small over ripe bananas

⅔ cup unbleached, all-purpose flour

½ tsp. baking soda

¼ tsp. sea salt

¼ cup plain soy milk yogurt

⅓ cup sugar

¼ cup walnuts

¼ cup vegetable oil

½ tsp. pure vanilla extract

Directions:

Combine the flour, baking soda, and salt in a bowl.

In a small bowl, mix the yoghurt, bananas, sugar, vegetable oil and vanilla extract.

Combine the wet ingredients with the dry. Don't over mix, just combine until well mixed. Fold in the walnuts at this stage.

Preheat the air fryer on 330 degrees Fahrenheit for 3 minutes

While the air fryer is preheating, pour half the batter into one loaf pan and the other half into a second loaf pan.

If you have a large (6-quart) air fryer, transfer the loaf pans to the air fryer basket

Air fry the banana bread at 330 degrees Fahrenheit for 20 - 22 minutes. They are done when a cake tester inserted into the loaves comes out clean.

Transfer the pans to a wire rack to cool for 30 minutes, before removing from the pans and serving.

314. Quinoa Carrot Cake

Servings: 6

Preparation Time: 5 mins

Cooking Time: 7 mins

Ingredients:

1½ cups cooked white quinoa

½ cup uncooked quinoa

¼ cup coconut flour

½ cup cooked carrot puree

1 cup freshly grated carrots

3 tbsp. flaxmeal in 8 tbsp. water (allow to gel for 5 minutes)

1 tsp. baking soda

1 tsp. baking powder

1 tsp. cinnamon

½ tsp. nutmeg

½ tsp. ground ginger

2 tbsp. blackstrap molasses

Raisins, to taste

Directions:

Combine all the ingredients at once in a large bowl and mix well. Coat a baking dish with coconut oil and pour in the cake batter.

Bake in the air fryer at 350 degrees Fahrenheit for 7 minutes.

Once done, let the cake cool and, if desired, frost with vegan cream cheese frosting.

315. Boston Cream Doughnuts

Servings: 12

Preparation Time: 3 hrs.

Cooking Time: 5 mins

Ingredients:

For the dough:

¾ cup soy milk, warmed to 65 degrees Fahrenheit

1 tbsp. flax meal

1 tbsp. dry yeast

3 tbsp. hot water

1 tbsp. vegan granulated sugar

2½ cup all-purpose flour

½ tsp. baking powder

¼ tsp. salt

⅛ tsp. cardamom

⅛ tsp. nutmeg

2½ cups peanut oil

4 tbsp. vegan butter or coconut oil

For the Custard:

1½ cups soy milk

1 tbsp. vegan butter

¼ cup granulated sugar + 1 tbsp. more

4 tbsp. cornstarch

A pinch of turmeric, only for color

1 tsp. pure vanilla extract

For the Glaze:

1½ tbsp. agave nectar

4 tbsp. coconut oil

5 tbsp. cocoa powder

For the Sprinkles:

1½ cup icing sugar

1 tbsp. water

1 tsp. vanilla extract

A pinch of salt

Food color, as needed

Directions:

For the Dough:

Sprinkle dry yeast over the warm milk and allow to prove for 5 minutes until the yeast begins to sponge.

Melt the vegan butter and then combine the flax meal with hot water. Let it stand to gel for 5 - 10 minutes

In a mixer fitted with a dough hook combine all the ingredients including the yeast-milk mixture (except for the oil).

Mix on a low speed until everything is well mixed; about 30 seconds.

Scrape the bottom and sides of the mixer bowl to help the dough along and mix on a low to medium speed for 8 minutes on medium speed.

Place the dough into a lightly oiled bowl and let rise in a warm spot, covered, for 30 minutes

Fold the dough onto itself and continue to prove for a further 30 minutes.

Turn the dough out onto a clean lightly floured surface and roll it to be a quarter to half an inch thick

Cut the dough with a 3 inch heart shaped cookie cutter

Transfer the donuts to a baking parchment lined sheet pan and allow the doughnuts to rest for a further 30-45 minutes.

Brush the donuts lightly with oil and fry at 400 degrees Fahrenheit for 10 minutes, until golden.

For the Custard:

Combine all the ingredients except for the vanilla extract and butter in a medium sauce pan over a medium to high heat. Bring to the boil stirring constantly.

Once bubbling be sure to stir constantly to avoid burning on the bottom of the pan, and let boil on a low heat for 30 seconds.

Add the vanilla extract and vegan butter. Stir to melt the butter

Pour into a shallow dish and cover with cling film to avoid a skin forming and, then refrigerate until cold.

For the Glaze:

Combine all ingredients for the glaze together in a small sauce pan and heat on a low heat, stirring constantly, until melted. Set aside.

For the Sprinkles:

Combine all the ingredients for the glaze together and stir to form a stiff dough.

Add the desired food color and fill the donuts.

Serve and enjoy!

316. Semolina Cake

Servings: 6

Preparation Time: 30 mins

Cooking Time: 30 mins

Ingredients:

1 cup fine farina, milled fine

2 cups hot water

1 cup dried fruit

1 cup sugar

1 cup almond milk

¼ cup soy yogurt

¼ cup coconut oil

1 tsp. ground cardamom

½ tsp. baking soda

1 tsp. baking powder

Directions:

Soak the dried fruit in hot water and set aside.

Grease an 8-inch heat-safe baking pan and keep aside.

In a large mixing bowl whisk together the milk, farina, oil, sugar, soy yogurt and cardamom.

Set this mixture aside for 20 minutes to allow the farina to soften and absorb the liquid.

Drain the dried fruit well, and mix into the batter.

Add the baking soda and baking powder and mix well.

Pour the cake batter into the prepared cake pan and set the pan into the air fryer basket.

Set the air fryer to 330 degrees Fahrenheit for 25 minutes.

At the end of the bake time, insert a cake tester to check for doneness. It should come out clean.

Remove the pan, let rest for 10 minutes and then unmold the cake.

Serve and enjoy!

Chapter 9 21 Day Meal Plan

DAY	BREAKFAST	MAINS	SNACK/DESSERT
1.	Cranberry Coconut Quinoa	Crispy Ranch Potatoes	Chocolate Cookies
2.	Sweet Quinoa Mix	Roasted Vegetables	Simple And Sweet Bananas
3.	Chia Pudding	Stewed Okra	Coffee Pudding
4.	Simple Creamy Breakfast Potatoes	Healthy Summer Vegetables	Almond And Vanilla Cake
5.	Sweet Potatoes Mix	Tasty Ranch Potatoes	Blueberry Cake
6.	Breakfast Bowls	Easy Dill Carrots	Peach Cobbler
7.	Hot Polenta Rounds	Delicious Fruit Salsa	Easy Pears Dessert
8.	Breakfast-Style Potatoes	Creamy Sweet Potato Mash	Sweet Strawberry Mix
9.	Roasted Tofu Broccoli Bowl With Quinoa	Ranch Carrots	Sweet Bananas And Sauce
10.	Air-Grilled Tomatoes	Perfect Mashed Potatoes	Raspberry Bars
11.	Mediterranean Chickpeas Breakfast	Herb Lentil Rice Veggie Quinoa	Sweetened Plantains

12.	Pumpkin Breakfast Muffins	Spicy Rice	Baked Apples With Pumpkin Spice
13.	Delicious Porridge	Sweet Carrots	Vegan Brownies
14.	Strawberry Quinoa	Sweetcorn Risotto	Berry Crumble
15.	Breakfast Broccoli And Tofu Bowls	Refried Pinto Beans	Apple Chips
16.	Cinnamon Oatmeal	Spicy Rice	Fruit Kebab
17.	French Fries	Easy Cilantro Lime Rice	Fruit Crumble
18.	Potato Hash	Indian Potato Curry	Cocoa Berries Cream
19.	Coconut Rice	Smooth Mashed Potatoes	Lemon Cream
20.	Cool Tofu Breakfast Mix	Delicious Chickpea Hummus	Easy Buns
21.	Cranberry Coconut Quinoa	Banana Oatmeal	Easy Blackberries Scones

Conclusion

Air Fryers have now become popular in many of the households especially because it is a great alternative to deep frying that too with much less oil. And if you have chosen to begin cooking your family meals in an air fryer than this complete guide is definitely going to help you getting started.

After reading through the incredible benefits of the air fryer and browsing through the wide range of recipes outlined, am sure you must be waiting to get your hands on your air fryer.

Good luck on this new journey of Air fryer style cooking!

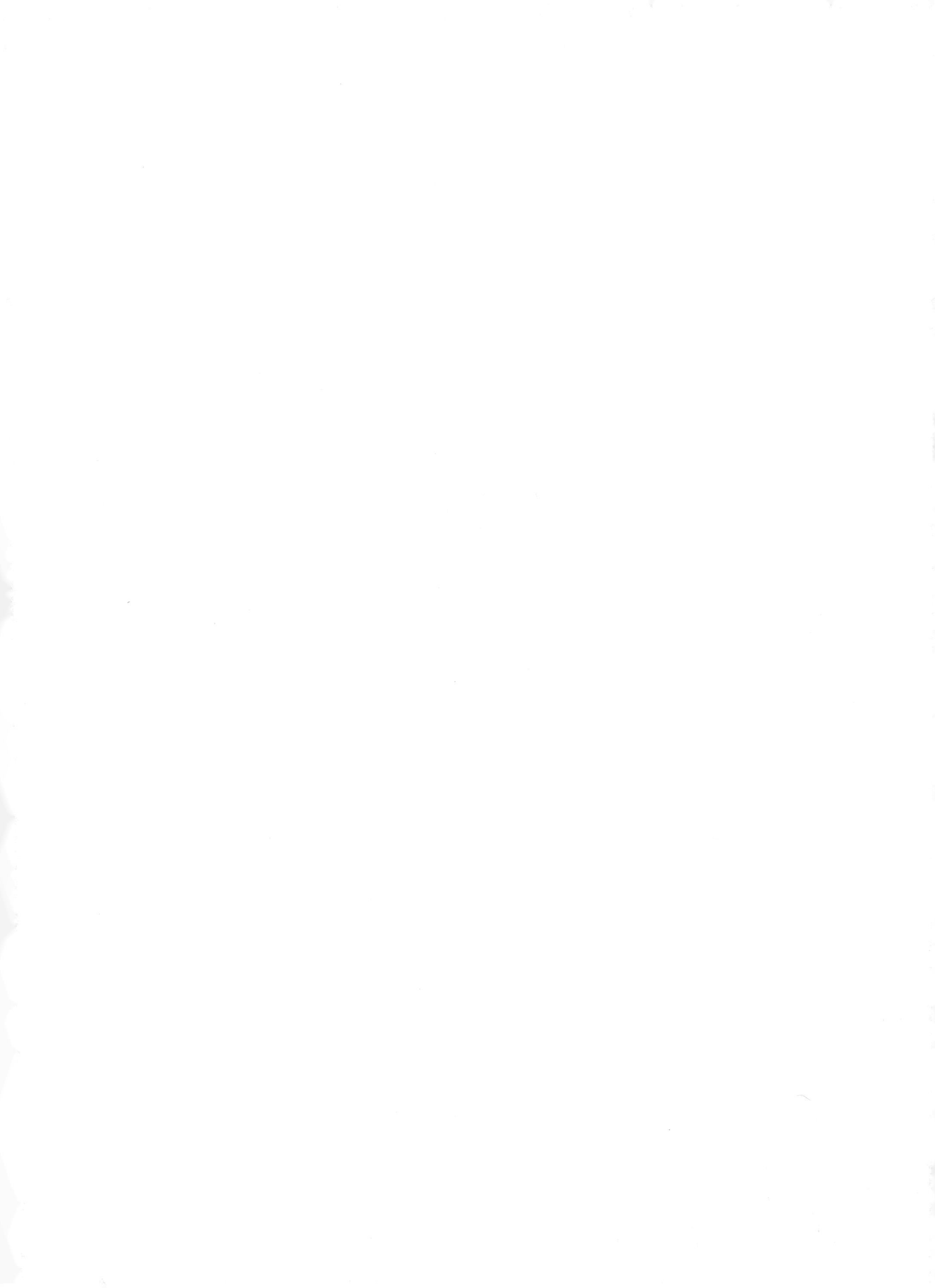